Passive Smoking and Cardiovascular Pathology: Mechanisms and Physiopathological Bases of Damage

PASSIVE SMOKING AND CARDIOVASCULAR PATHOLOGY: MECHANISMS AND PHYSIOPATHOLOGICAL BASES OF DAMAGE

AURELIO LEONE

Nova Science Publishers, Inc.
New York

For permission to use material from this book please contact us:
Telephone 631-231-7269; Fax 631-231-8175
Web Site: http://www.novapublishers.com

Library of Congress Cataloging-in-Publication Data

Leone, Aurelio.

Passive smoking and cardiovascular pathology : mechanisms and physiopathological bases of damage / Aurelio Leone.

p. ; cm.

Includes bibliographical references and index.

ISBN-13: 978-1-60021-644-2 (hardcover)

ISBN-10: 1-60021-644-7 (hardcover)

1. Smoking--Physiological effect. 2. Passive smoking--Physiological effect. 3. Cardiovascular system--Pathophysiology. 4. Heart--Diseases. I. Title.

[DNLM: 1. Cardiovascular Diseases--etiology. 2. Tobacco Smoke Pollution--adverse effects. WG 120 L583p 2007]

RA1242.T6L46 2007

613.85--dc22

2007005743

Published by Nova Science Publishers, Inc. ✢ New York

CONTENTS

PREFACE

To my grandchildren
Elena and Aurelio;
to Elena, my sweet wife.

One could say —"the millionth book concerning tobacco!" It may be yes! But if authors, editors, social educators continue to debate such a subject, it means that there is a need and the tobacco problem is so far to be solved.

However, the contents of the present volume is not a systematic treatment of what it has been written on tobacco and the heart, but a focus mainly of the reliable results on the relationship between passive smoking and cardiovascular pathology.

Indeed, findings concerning the harmful effects of passive smoking, namely isolated or public exposure to someone else's smoking, on individuals' health have begun approximately in the seventh decade, and the progression in studies slow at first but has been followed by an effective increase of scientific reports in the years after.

Deriving from that, it could seem that a custom phenomenon involved passive smoking findings. Indeed, that is not true since beginning observations provided interesting results of potential damage due to environmental tobacco smoke for those individuals who underwent its exposure and this occurence stimulated several researchers to intensify their findings on the subject.

Aerial inhalation of toxic vapors containing some of those components which are present in sidestream smoking were known to be harmful for the health in circumstances which were different from smoking exposure. These components such as ammonia, nitrosamines, benzene and its metabolites were responsible of acute or chronic toxicity for those people who were working particularly in public spaces thet were used, in past times, for washing and iron clothes. Reports identified acute and chronic symptoms of poisoning from aforesaid inhaled vapors with a major incidence in Chinese ironing women.

Once more, the knowledge of the damages from acute or chronic toxicity due to carbon monoxide, which is one of the most important component of passive smoking, goes back to the beginning of time. Therefore, it is astonishing that a lack of attention has been placed on the harmful effects of passive smoking that was recognized to have toxic chemicals with already well known negative effects on the health.

However, this gap has been filled, as above said, by flourishing findings that have demonstrated, undoubtedly, confirmation of a heavy harm to individuals' health with a clear major incidence for cardiovascular system and of the lungs.

The author of this book occupies an important position on the findings concerning the relationship between cardiovascular pathology and passive smoking since he came to study the problem in the seventh decade. Today cardiovascular damage from smoking is known as theorem of Leone. It may be formulated as follows: "Active smoking injures the cardiovascular system chronically, causing structural lesions, which become, in the long run, irreversible alterations mainly related to coronary atherosclerosis. In contrast, passive smoking causes transiently impaired cardiac performance which may be considerably harmful for those people with established ischaemic heart disease". At the end of this book, this theorem will be discussed again briefly to show that increasing findings overtake such a statement.

This book reflects the current views on the relationship between cardiovascular pathology and passive smoking, providing the main achievements obtained with the findings on the subject. Therefore, I believe that the book can provide information for up to date physicians, researchers, students, and legislators on the state of art of a research area that is continuously in growth.

Aurelio Leone

Chapter 1

CHARACTERISTIC OF PASSIVE SMOKING

ABSTRACT

The knowledge of those factors able to influence the characteristics of passive smoking has to be borne in mind in order to assess the causes of damage due to environmental tobacco smoke is caused.

Of tobacco culture, there is to recognize the leaf shape like a "cupule" has to be recognized as well as the distribution of water and alkaloids. Also, the different types of tobacco manufacturing can provide useful information on the characteristics of passive smoking.

Both active smoking and passive smoking contain the same chemical compounds although they are in lower concentrations in passive smoking. However, the major length of time exposure for passive smoking, particular mixing of chemical compounds, types of environment, and health conditions of exposed people, may impair heavily the action of passive smoking.

Finally, four types of studies assess the damage due to passive smoking exposure on an individuals' health: clinical studies, epidemiological studies, combined clinical and epidemiological studies, and experimental studies. These studies, all together, provide a good confirmation of the risk due to passive smoking exposure, even if experimental studies are those which undoubtedly demonstrate the existence of the damage.

Keywords: Passive smoking: characteristics, tobacco, culture, manufacturing, tobacco chemicals, environment, lifestyle, health.

Passive smoking, also named involuntary smoking, environmental tobacco smoking, secondhand smoking, is inhaled by both smokers and nonsmokers with similar health effects in some occurences and different responses in others.

Understanding the effects and mechanisms able to cause damage on individuals' health needs some knowledge that involve different conditions, the main of which, are listed in table 1.1. The analysis of these factors provide rudiments as well as set the characteristics of passive smoking.

Table 1.1. Main factors to be known for understanding passive smoking characteristics

1.	Tobacco plant and its leaves
2.	Tobacco leaves manufacturing
3.	Same chemical compounds of active and passive smoking
4.	Differences in chemical compound action for active and passive smoking
5.	Environment
6.	Lifestyle of exposed individuals
7.	Health of exposed individuals
8.	Type of studies related to passive smoking

This chapter will focus on those points of Table 1 that may influence the mechanisms of passive smoking as well as its characteristics.

1.1. AND 1.2. TOBACCO PLANT AND ITS LEAVES

Tobacco [1–2], firstly cultivated by the Indians of North and South America, is the name attributed to the plant and its leaves and flowers (Figures 1.1. and 1.2.) of different species of Nicotiana of the Solanaceae family . It may be used immediately fresh, but it is more often used after manufacturing to prepare tobacco products for smoking. The plant, fresh leaves of which are used to be chewed, is the Nicotiana rustica. Manufactured tobacco for smoking makes use of Nicotiana tabacum. Leaf surface contains a large amount of alkaloids abounding particularly in nicotine. On the contrary, tobacco flowers (Figure 1.2.) are rich of vegetal oils which are mainly used for soap and paint industries.

The particular shape of the leaves associated with soil moisture permits to clarify some important characteristics which need to be considered to go into details of the acting mechanism concerning passive smoking.

When tobacco leaf is used as chewing, only alkaloids abounding in nicotine and similar components are absorbed without presence of carbon monoxide or other chemicals which derive from burned tobacco. Otherwise, tobacco manipulated for smoking use undergoes some changes that permit it to damage individuals' health in many different ways and by action of different toxic chemicals. Some of these chemicals are similar for active smokers and passive smokers, although they usually act with different concentrations. Cut plants or pulled leaves are immediately stored into tobacco barns where they will be cured. This process produces a degradation of the carotenoids in tobacco leaves by a slow oxidation that provides an aromatic flavor particularly agreable for the smokers.

Three common methods of curing are used for tobacco treatment (Table 1.2): curing by air, fire, and flue.

Air-curing is accomplished primarily in buildings equipped with ventilators. Often tomes, coke, charcoal or liquid petroleum gas are used to provide artificial heat necessary, in any cases, to "help" natural conditions. The time required for air-curing varies from one to two months.

The fire-curing process is similar to that used for air-curing but open wood fires are kindled on the dirt floor of the barn and not in a building after the tobacco has been hanging from two to six days, so that the smoke amalgamates with the leaves. This procedure provides a typical creosote aroma. The firing process may be continuous or intermittent from three weeks to as long as ten weeks until curing is complete and tobacco leaves reach the desired characteristics.

Finally, in the third method of tobacco curing, flue-cured tobacco is originally strung onto tobacco sticks, which are hung from tier-poles in large cubital barns. This method also needs firing. For firing, fuels used are wood, coal, oil and liquid petroleum gas.

The different time that may be necessary for tobacco curing depends either from the type of curing used, or in presence of the same method of curing, by very little differences in plants of tobacco arising in different countries.

Table 1.2. Common methods of curing for tobacco leaves

Method	Leaf Storage
Air-curing	Ventilated Buildings
Fire-curing	Dirt floor Barns
Flue-curing	Large cubital Barns

When curing process is performed, particularly under heat chemical and physical changes occur in the tobacco leaves. An added major concentration in toxic chemicals that influence the characteristics of passive smoking are the result of such a process.

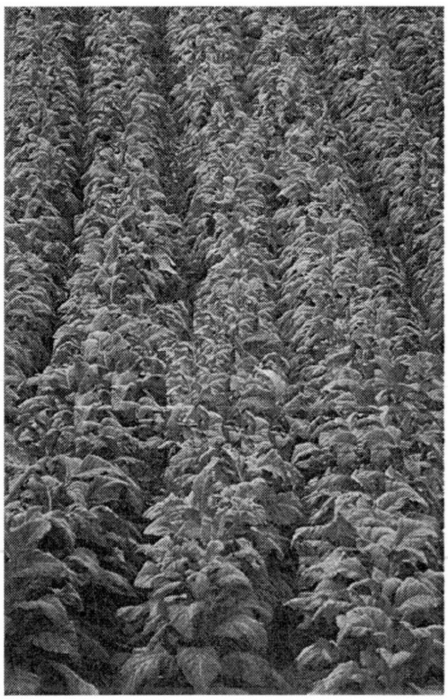

Figure 1.1. Plants of Nicotiana tabacum native from South America are usually used in commerce for industrial use. The particular type of leaves with a characteristic shape like a "cupule" can be observed. Such a shape is necessary to ensure a uniform and diffuse distribution of water and chemical components along the entire leaf. Soluble alkaloids, therefore, are present along the entire leaf and their extraction is almost complete. Nicotine, which is a compound highly soluble in water, follows these characteristics up to a level beyond which further extraction is not possible. However, high doses of the alkaloid may be usually extracted.

As already desribed, tobacco plant flowers are used by chemical and not tobacco industries to prepare particularly paints. However, flowers too may exert toxic effects.

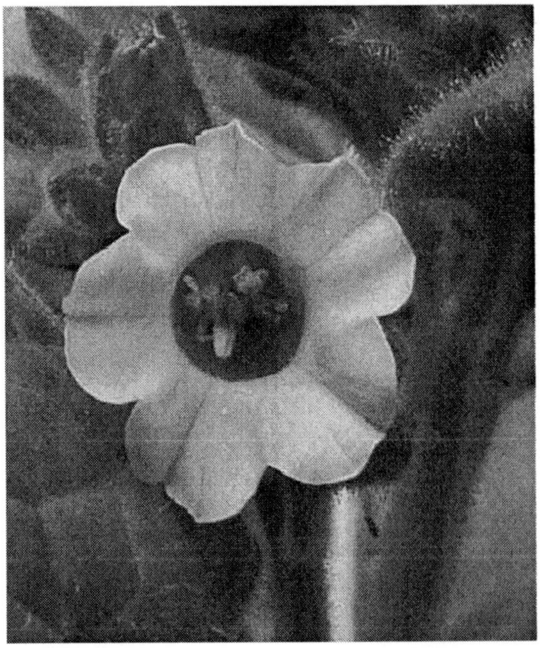

Figure 1.2. Tobacco flower with its buds.

What has been described until now about the culture and manufacturing tobacco leaves could seem to have a small impact on understanding the characteristics of passive smoke. Really, this is not how matters stand. The knowledge of the structure and manufacture of tobacco plant provides basic rudiments to establish exactly the potential damage determined by passive smoking. Indeed, an example of passive intoxication from tobacco fresh leaves, but not smoked tobacco, was described among Indian tobacco harvesters [3]. Workers can absorb nicotine through the skin, often resulting in nausea, vomiting and weakness. Workers without gloves reported symptoms and had a significantly higher excretion of nicotine and cotinine than controls who used gloves. However, gloves reduced symptoms and urinary excretion of nicotine and cotinine although their use did not completely protect those harvesters who dressed the gloves. This clinical study demonstrated that nicotine in fresh leaves is well absorbed through the skin and skin protection in tobacco harvesters can reduce, but not avoid, completely toxic symptoms.

Moreover, some other facts should be considered.

Tobacco fresh leaves, because of their shape, size, chemical compounds, and water, burn by producing much less carbon monoxide than that produced by cured tobacco leaves. Moreover, the paper, which rolls up the cigarettes, plays a basic role for the release of toxic chemicals because of its burning. That increases in amount toxic residuum of passive smoking, particularly carbon monoxide that usually causes a significant damage to cardiovascular system and lungs [4].

This fact should be considered carefully when passive smoking characteristics (sidestream) are analyzed, although, even nowdays, several scientific papers do not follow this way and consequently, different results are reached. Furthermore, manufacturing tobacco, whatever method is used, causes grinding and drying up leaves, and which causes a significant change in leak water in burning volume. With their remarkable increase, that will influence the concentration of passive smoking components. Then, increased concentration of some compounds causes higher condensing of residuum in passive smoking with difference in composition with regard to those of active smoking. Therefore, a concise knowledge of tobacco culture, storage and manufacturing is a useful fact in order to understand passive smoking characteristics as well as its mechanisms of damage that differs, and in some cases considerably differs, from that caused by active smoking.

Fresh tobacco, active smoking and passive smoking absorption have differences which must be kept in mind. Chemical properties of fresh and burned tobacco particularly should be kept in mind with some compounds. Moreover, chemicals contained in environmental tobacco smoke may aggregate other air pollutants and, by doing so, potentiate their harmful effects.

1.3. Chemical Compounds of Active and Passive Smoking

Both active and passive smoke have a chemical composition that will be analyzed in detail in the next chapter. However, in view of the influence that tobacco chemistry may have on passive smoking characteristics, concise news will be given in the present subdivision. Some tobacco chemicals are those basic factors which cause damage to cardiovascular system.

Adverse effects on heart and vessels are mediated through the action of many chemical compounds that are concentrated and condensed into tobacco mixture [5]. Over 4,000 chemicals have been identified in smoke and a large majority of these have carcinogenic and/or negative cardiovascular effects in humans and animals. Animal findings, until now considered as findings on animals exposed to active smoking action, really should be explained as an indirect exposure to cigarette smoke in a large majority of cases, and then, the damage observed has to be seen as damage due to passive exposure.

Three main smoking markers (Table 1.3.) are usually studied as an indicator of both active and passive smoke exposure in epidemiological surveys [6–7] on heart and blood vessels because of their toxicity and laboratory assessment. Their harmful effects on cardiovascular system are, however, including those determined by other possible chemicals of passive smoking which, on the contrary, characterize mainly other organs.

These components, when absorbed into the blood, act like free or bound plasma constituents and have a different half-life that is about 5 hours for carbon monoxide when it is bound to hemoglobin, 16 hours for cotinine, and 6.5 days for thiocyanates.

Although inhaled after tobacco manufacturing and burning, but not in fresh leaves, carbon monoxide plays a basic role in long-term damage from both active smoking and passive smoking. Nicotine intoxication may also occur and depends on both fresh tobacco exposure and exposure to active or passive smoking. Thiocyanate toxicity is too hard to establish since different foods, which are rich in these substances, may adulterate and confuse obtained responses.

Many other chemicals, as already said, may negatively influence heart and blood vessels, but their action is limited when compared to that due to carbon monoxide, nicotine and thiocyanate. On the contrary, these other chemicals, such as ammonia, benzene, 2-naphtylamine, nitrosamines, benzoanthracene and benzopyrene [8] contained in a greater amount in passive smoking – sidestream smoke – have prevailingly heavy carcinogenic effects.

Table 1.3. Chemical compounds able to cause cardiovascular damage from active and passive smoking

Chemicals	Site
1. Nicotine and its metabolites (particularly Cotinine)	Fresh tobacco leaves
	Active smoking
	Passive smoking
2. Carbon monoxide	Active smoking
	Passive smoking
3. Thiocyanate	Fresh tobacco leaves
	Active smoking
	Passive smoking

1.4. Difference in Chemical Compounds for Active and Passive Smoke

As previously described, essentially similar composition characterizes active and passive smoke. However, some differences exist between the two types, either for that concerning component chemical phase or for their concentration and mechanism of acting. There is poor emphasis given to that in different studies. Therefore, a question arises: is the smoke inhaled actively, as smoking a cigarette, different from that due to passive smoking exposure?

Both types of smoking, active smoking and passive smoking, contain thousands of toxic chemicals which have almost similar characteristics, although their concentration varies widely. Changes in concentration depend from the number of cigarettes smoked, amount of passive smoke residuum, type and structure of the environments, individual's smoking pattern.

Another factor to be considered is the duration of exposure to smoking that is short in active smokers (about 2 minutes for each smoked cigarette) but longer in those individuals who are exposed to passive smoke, since cigarette end continues to exhale toxic substances into the environment for a long period of time. Moreover, such a fact involves inhalation of carbon monoxide which is a compound of burned tobacco but not fresh tobacco. Therefore, the higher chemical concentration absorbed by active smoking is partially balanced from the longer duration of exposure to passive smoking [9]. This longer time of exposure to smoke residuum may be responsible for an effective mixture and chemical combination among the different toxic products with changes which determine difference, in the long run, in the type of constituents of active and passive smoke. Mixing of environmental smoke is a consequence of gaseous and steam phase of tobacco chemicals which have moving particles. They may aggregate or break away and that depends strongly on their concentration and temperature into passive smoke residuum. Therefore, environmental tobacco smoke consists of a dynamic mixture in ambient air, the concentration and composition of which vary widely because of their physical phase. This dynamic process will determine differences in chemical compounds and their concentration between active and passive smoke as well as difficulty to quantify the exact level of damage caused by passive smoking unless in those cases where study methods are carefully standardized. Such a condition makes extremely hard to interpret correctly epidemiological data, whereas, on the contrary, experimental studies may provide much more reproducible results [10] when they meet experimentally similar procedures.

Three main phases characterize passive smoking (Table 1.4.): sidestream smoke which is defined as the smoke that drifts from the end of the lit cigarette, mainstream smoke , which is the smoke inhaled directly through the burning cigarette by the smokers, and the exhaled mainstream smoke which is the smoke breathed out by the smoker from their lungs. Also the composition of mainstream smoke and exhaled mainstream smoke can likely differ since some of the compounds in smoke are retained by the smokers or otherwise altered by the process of combustion and, then, exhaled smoking. Indeed, these factors influence heavily passive smoking characteristics.

Table 1.4. Main phases which characterize passive smoking and their chemicals

Type of smoking	Chemicals
1. Sidestream smoke (the smoke that drifts from the end of the lit cigarette)	Carbon monoxide
	Nicotine
	Carcinogens (polynuclear hydrocarbons, aromatic amines, nitrosamines, tar, benzopyrene, vinyl-chloride)
2. Mainstream smoke (inhaled by smoked cigarette)	Nicotine
	Carbon monoxide
	Aromatic amines
	Nitrosamines
	Benzopyrene
	Naphtlylamine
	Benzoanthracene
3. Exhaled mainstream smoke (breathed out by smoker)	Carbon monoxide
	Carcinogens
	Nicotine (lower concentration)

The particles of sidestream smoke are smaller than those of mainstream smoke, meaning that they can be inhaled more deeply into the lungs [11].

Then, once the smoke has left the cigarette, its physical nature and relative chemical composition will change dramatically since its particles evaporate rapidly or condense according to some characteristics of the environment, particularly its level of pollution due to other chemical pollutants which strengthen the power of smoking ambient pollutants.

Although tobacco smoke, as aforesaid, consists of many thousands of toxic chemicals, the greatest mass of smoke is due to carbon dioxide, carbon monoxide and water [12–13] containing soluble toxics particularly nicotine and thiocyanate. Many of the other components have such a low concentration in environmental tobacco smoke or dosed by using very expensive sophisticated techniques that provide results of poor significance.

Studies conducted in human nonsmokers exposed to passive smoke, dose measurable levels of nicotine or cotinine and carbon monoxide in the blood [14–17], with an incidence up to 90 percent of exposed subjects.

1.5. Environment

Among those factors, which are prevailing to influence the cardiovascular damage due to passive smoking exposure, the environment undoubtedly plays a strong role with regard to the wide variety of its physico-chemical characteristics. Therefore, even if a detailed description of the different properties of the environment is not the main purpose of this book, some points of view are necessary to discuss a better focus on passive smoking

Architecturally and hygienically, an environment is a complex structure that involves individuals and all living organisms modifying, determining and organizing particularly some events of their life or characters. However, the natural environment, that should be relatively unaffected by human activity, really does not exist. Humans must live in a polluted environment where different factors act to cause pollution. Many industrial activities as well, contribute to an individuals' lifestyle to negatively change.

Many of these substances arise from cigarette smoking exposure. The level of some smoke constituents in the environmental tobacco smoke depends (Table 1.5.) approximately on the environment space, ventilation rate, decay rate, mixing rate, and room volume as well as number of cigarettes smoked into the environment, number of nonsmoker people present and concomitant presence or absence of active smokers.

Table 1.5. Factors influencing the level of smoking constituents in environment

1. Environment characteristics	environment space
	ventilation rate
	decay rate
	mixing rate
	room volume
2. Number of smoked cigarettes	
3. Number of living people	
4. Presence or absence of active smokers	

Environment space is one of the most determinant factor for identifying cardiovascular damage due to passive smoking exposure. Exposure to environmental tobacco smoke [18] may occur everywhere but particularly in the home, in the workplace, in social settings, and in public places. Measurements of environmental tobacco smoke concentrations [19–32] showed a strong interest for researchers for those in the offices, restaurants, bars, public places and less for those in home probably because of difficulties due to family reasons. Figure 3 shoes evidence of percent distribution of measurements carried out in the different seats.

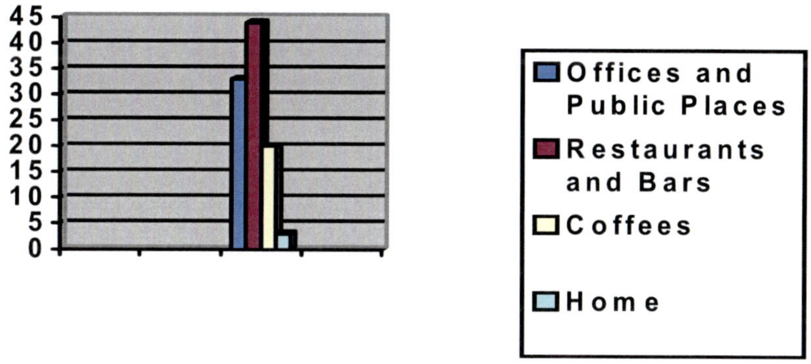

Figure 1.3. Percent environment places analysed for passive smoking measurements.

An important role in determining indoor and/or outdoor pollution plays the degree of ambient ventilation. This parameter widely varies since it is influenced by natural factors or architectural criteria as well as a number of living people.

Open spaces usually have lower concentrations of toxic chemicals due to passive smoking since these substances are distributed and diluted in a larger mass of air atmosphere, although the global pollution of the area may be influenced by possible presence of other pollution sources. Really, there are many sources of indoor pollutants in both gaseous and/or particulate phases which derive from industrial buildings, fires, car motors, and so on. An effective ventilation may help particularly indoor spaces. Ambient concentrations of environmental tobacco smoke products have been measured in different ways. A mean of passive smoking chemicals [24] concerning seats where both nonsmokers and smokers were living gave indoor nicotine concentrations of 3.2 micrograms/cubic metre, carbon monoxide of 2.3 ppm, ammonia from 1,000 to 4,500 micrograms/cubic metre, particulate from 55 to 96 mg/cubic metre. However, efforts are conducted to limit environmental tobacco smoke exposure or build spaces effectively protected.

Decay rate is also a parameter to be considered to establish the potential hazard of passive smoking to the environment and then to the health of individuals. While on the one hand, toxic chemical decay may reduce environment concentration, on the other hand, mixing of decomposed compounds could develop or potentiate the harmful effects that chemicals have. It has also been obesrved that all chemical changes of passive smoke compounds are influenced by thousands of unpredictable factors which, in the large majority of cases, can alter their concentration so that the true level of harm often escapes whatever assessment.

Finally, room volume is a parameter that is strongly related to the above factors. It has a basic role not only to establish epidemiologically the potential harm which may result from tobacco chemical concentrations, but also provide reproducible data in those experimental studies [10, 33] that have been conducted in structures with similar capacity.

Obviously, the number of people who are living in an environment, as well as the number of active smokers and, smoked cigarettes, particularly influence the environmental characteristics and, consequently, the responses related to the effects of passive smoking. As one can deduce, these factors can provide absolutely different results since they depend on a large number of variables not ditrectly related to the environment.

1.6. Lifestyle of Exposed Individuals

The first step to choice for a healthy lifestyle of nonsmokers would be to persuade active smokers not to smoke. Furtherly, educational programs to inform people to avoid the deleterious effects of every type of smoking must be strongly conducted to reach effective results. And, in this way, many antismoking campaigns are in progress.

A correct lifestyle is fundamental to ensure both better physiologic response of human body and, particularly, prevent a large number of diseases with significant reduction in mortality, morbidity and permanent disability of living subjects [4, 17, 34]. Lifestyle is a major modifiable parameter to reduce the incidence of adverse events.

It is well documented that avoiding passive smoking exposure and going in for physical activity [35] reduce cardiovascular risk of recurrent cardiovascular events with a statistically significant incidence. Moreover, a correct lifestyle alone, in case of exposure to passive smoking, could reduce the harmful impact due to environmental tobacco smoke in those people who follow such recommendations.

Presence of cardiovascular risk factors in young people have been researched [36–37]. A correct lifestyle, avoiding sedentary life, could change these patterns.

A free smoking atmosphere would be the ideal result to improve individuals' lifestyle and then reduce the harmful effects due to passive smoking exposure, which is more and more considered as a major risk factor for cardiovascular events or even an etiologic factor of heart diseases [38–42], as it will be described later.

Therefore, an effective change in lifestyle to fight passive smoking exposure may be carried out (Table 1.6.) with absolute measures, avoiding total smoking exposure or relative measures consisting of reduced smoking exposure accompanied by regular physical activity and diet supplementation.

Table 1.6. Changes in lifestyle to fight passive smoking

1. Absolute measures	Avoid totally smoking exposure
2. Relative measures	Reduce passive smoking exposure
	Physical activity
	Diet supplementation (Vitamin C, Vitamin E, Antioxidants)

It has been well demonstrated [43] that a correct behaviour in following relative measures may decrease cardiovascular risk. Efforts then must be conducted attempting to put these measures into action.

1.7. Health of Exposed Individuals

This subdivision seats the goal to clarify the relationship between passive smoking and health of exposed people in an attempt to establish those altered changes of health that influence the characteristics of action as well as the mechanisms through which environmental tobacco smoke may increase cardiovascular damage. Treating cardiovascular pathology will be excluded here since it will be a basic subject of the next chapters.

The main parameter to analyze for establishing health of an individual who risks to be exposed to passive smoking is the oxygen saturation (figure 1.4.).

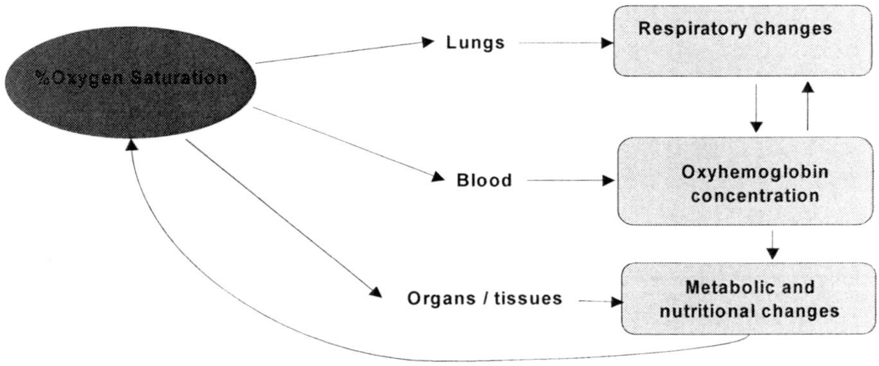

Figure 1.4. Physiologic role of oxygen saturation and its relationship with body organs. Percent (%) oxygen saturation influences the characteristics of respiratory changes which are related to oxyhemoglobin concentration; it provides metabolic and nutritional materials to body organs and tissues. From time to time, peripheral metabolic requests are the stimulus that regulates the percent oxygen saturation.

All those pathologic events that directly or indirectly influence the mechanisms of oxygen saturation level have to be examined since different percentages of oxygen saturation determine different responses to chemical compounds of passive smoking. Therefore, a large series of systemic pathologies as well as those subclinical conditions which need an improvement in oxygen saturation can be impaired as a response to passive smoking.

Particularly, carbon monoxide and all those smoke components defined generically as carcinogens influence oxygen saturation and then some specific diseases. On the contrary, nicotine and cotinine which are those smoke metabolites specifically used to determine environmental tobacco smoke exposure [16] of people are mainly related to functional cardiovascular events.

Adverse effects due to main compounds of passive smoking concern respiratory system, blood, immune function with regard to T-cells and antibody response which particularly feel the alterations in oxygen saturation and metabolism [44–48].

Among the main constituents of passive smoking, since nicotine plays its action particularly on adrenergic system and then it follows the way of cardiovascular metabolism and vessel function, carbon monoxide and carcinogens cause alterations of the aforesaid systems. Specifically, respiratory system and blood are closely related to oxygen saturation.

Both chronic and acute respiratory diseases are the result of a prolonged passive smoking exposure [49–53]. Exposure to tobacco smoke is one of the major causes of developing and then triggering an asthma attack. Moreover, further studies are showing an impaired lung function in those exposed people when they are compared to unexposed never smokers [54–55].

Passive smoking is also irritant for an individual's eyes and nose and can exacerbate respiratory symptoms particularly in children [44, 46–47].

Three characteristic mechanisms potentiate environmental tobacco smoke harm in respiratory diseases (Table 1.7.): the alterations of respiratory changes into the lungs, increased levels of carboxyhemoglobin due to carbon monoxide of environmental smoke, and reduced concentration of oxyhemoglobin into the blood as a consequence of the stronger linkage between carbon monoxide and hemoglobin. As one can see, mechanisms capable to induce damage are related, initially, to physiological response changes of respiratory system , particularly in that structure supporting the weight of breathing as the lungs, and then, to those deputed to oxygen transport. Therefore, primary preventive measures against damage from passive smoking should start from lung level.

Table 1.7. Mechanisms from passive smoking impairing respiratory function

Mechanism	Triggered cause
1. Alteration of gas changes into the lungs	Structural changes of lungs due to respiratory disease
2. Increased carboxyhemoglobin	Carbon monoxide from passive smoking
3. Reduced blood oxyhemoglobin	Linkage between carbon monoxide and hemoglobin

There is evidence that also other toxics of passive smoking may potentiate the action of carbon monoxide with documentably carcinogenic effects [4]. Further evidence that carcinogens from passive smoking are inhalated into the lung is the dosage of a tobacco-specific lung carcinogen [56] from the urine of nonsmokers exposed to environmental tobacco smoke.

Among hematologic diseases, the different level of hypoxia, induced by the strong relationship between carbon monoxide and haemoglobin, could influence the degree of anemia for those people who are suffering so that minimum hemoglobin cutoff values should be adjusted for smokers to compensate for the masking effect of smoking on the detection of anemia [57]. Smoking is also a risk factor for myelodysplastic syndromes [58–61]. However, leukemia and lymphoma are not among those cancers traditionally associated with cigarette smoking [62]. Therefore, the certain association between passive smoking and "so-called" blood cancers need further studies. The mutagenic effects due to some components of passive smoking could activate triggering mechanisms blood cancers rather than a direct action of these chemical compounds on blood cells.

In conclusion, there is a strong evidence that exposure to passive smoking increases the risk of respiratory diseases particularly in children as well as lung cancer in adults. Evidence also indicates that all those conditions that interfere negatively with percent oxygen saturation may impair the action of passive smoking components.

1.8. Types of Studies Related to Passive Smoking

Four types of studies have been conducted to assess the relationship between passive smoking and people's health (Table 1.8.): clinical studies, epidemiological studies, combined clinical and epidemiological studies, and experimental studies. A large majority of these studies was concerning chronic exposure to tobacco smoke components particularly in workplaces, public places, and home (Figure 1.3.), whereas some others, often conducted by using experimental procedures, were performed after acute exposure.

Table 1.8. Types of studies conducted to assess passive smoking harm on individuals

1. Clinical studies	Conducted on patients who were exposed to passive smoking.
2. Epidemiological studies	Conducted on people living with active smokers.
1.3. Combined clinico-epidemiological studies	Conducted on patients and healthy people living with active smokers.
1.4. Experimental studies	Conducted with different experimental procedures after acute exposure to passive smoke of both humans and animals.

From the analysis of the Table 1.8, there is evidence of widely dissimilar material of study resulting in the inability to reach unanimous conclusions on this matter. However, a large series of excellent studies [33, 39–40, 63–72] seem to identify a risk for the health of those people who meet a prolonged exposure to environmental tobacco smoke.

Papers provide results that arise from clinical observations of nonsmokers who suffered from different diseases and had been exposed to environmental tobacco smoke. The correlation of the disease with passive smoking was the result of a statistically selected process which provided an effective evidence of the matter [73]. However, analyzed data were complying with people living in restricted areas like home, workplaces, public buildings and, therefore, they did not examin the whole population of the studied area. All people living in the same spaces, even if they did not live with smokers, would be studied to assess if they suffered from the same disease that affected nonsmokers, living with smokers and thus, whether passive smoke inhalation was a clinical occurence due to characteristics of that area. However, there is no doubdt that statistical significance concerning the relationship between passive smoking and health damage reached a range of acceptable risk in clinical findings.

Also, epidemiological findings have some documented limits. Indeed, a large majority of these findings provide data that are the result of individual responses to mailed questionnaires [74]. Thus, at least some investigations could understimate the risk due to passive smoke exposure, whereas other findings could overestimate the risk. However, through these papers there is true evidence that environmental tobacco smoke is a hazard for individuals health. Moreover, particularly epidemiological studies continue to be the backbone of the findings into problems related to passive smoking exposure.

Findings of epidemiological and clinical papers on damage of cardiovascular system, due to passive smoking, will be described more in detail in a later chapter.

Experimental findings demonstrate undoubtedly the harmful effects of passive smoking. Some papers also showed that the damage due to passive smoking is a reproducible [10] damage when the same experimental procedures are conducted.

Experimental studies have been conducted in both humans and animals by using different procedures of passive smoking exposure as well as different anatomical seats of investigations [33, 75–82]. Moreover, experimental studies permit one to understand the main mechanisms of damage, its pathological patterns, and biochemical characteristics of passive smoking.

REFERENCES

[1] Clayton EE, McMurtrey JE Jr. Tobacco diseases and their control. US Department of Agriculture; *Farmer's Bulletin.* 2023, 1950.

[2] Breen TH. *Tobacco culture. Source on tobacco culture in eighteenth-century Virginia.* Princeton University Press 1985; 46 – 55.

[3] Ghosh SK, Gokani VN, Doctor PB, Parikh JR, Kashyap SK. Intervention studies against "green symptoms" among Indian tobacco harvesters. *Arch. Environ. Health.* 1991; 46: 316 – 7.

[4] Peto R, Lopez AD, Boreham J, Thun M, Heath C. *Mortality from smoking in developed countries : 1950 – 2000.* Oxford: Oxford University Press 1994.

[5] Byrd JC. Environmental tobacco smoke: Medical and legal issues. *Medical Clinics of North America* 1992; 76: 377 – 97.

[6] Greenberg RA, Haley NJ, Ersel RA, Loda FA. Measuring the exposure of infants to tobacco smoke. *N. Engl. J. Med.* 1984; 310: 1075 – 8.

[7] Strachan DP, Jarvis MJ, Feyerabend C. Passive smoking, salivary cotinine concentration and middle ear effusion in 7-year old children. *Br. Med. J.* 1989; 289: 1549 – 52.

[8] Leone A, Giannini D, Bellotto C, Balbarini A. Passive smoking and coronary heart disease. *Current Vascular. Pharm.* 2004; 2: 175 – 82.

[9] Fielding JE, Phenow KJ. Health effects of involuntary smoking. *N. Engl. J. Med.* 1988; 319: 1452 – 60.

[10] Leone A. Cardiovascular damage from smoking: a fact or belief? *Int. J. Cardiol.* 1993; 38: 113 – 7.

[11] US Department of Health and Human Services. *The Health Consequences of Involuntary Smoking. A Report of the Surgeon General.* Rockville, Md, Centers for Disease Control, Center for Health Promotion and Education, Office on Smoking and Health. 1981; DHHS Publication N° (CDC) 87 – 8398.

[12] Sterling TD, Collet CW, Sterling EM. Environmental tobacco smoke and indoor air quality in modern office work environments. *J. Occup. Med.* 1987; 29: 57 – 61.

[13] Proctor CJ. The analysis of the contribution of ETS to indoor air. In *Indoor Ambient and Air Quality*, Perry R and Kirk PW, Selper Ltd, London 1988; 57 – 66.

[14] Jarvis MJ, Tunstall-Pedoe H, Feyerabend C, Vesey C, Saloojee Y. Comparison of tests used to distinguish smokers from nonsmokers. *Am. J. Public Health.* 1987; 77: 1435 – 8.

[15] Benowitz NL, Jacob P. Nicotine and cotinine elimination pharmacokinetics in smokers and non smokers. *Clin. Pharmacol. Ther.* 1993; 53: 316 – 23.

[16] Benowitz NL. Cotinine as a biomarker of environmental tobacco smoke exposure. *Epidemiol. Rev.* 1996; 18: 188 – 204.

[17] Leone A. Biochemical markers of cardiovascular damage from tobacco smoke. *Curr. Pharm. Design.* 2005; 11: 2199 – 2208.

[18] Pirkle JL, Flegal KM, Bernert JT, Brody DJ, Etzel RA, Maurer KR. Exposure of the US population to environmental tobacco smoke. The Third National Health and Nutrition Examination Survey, 1988 to 1991. *JAMA.* 1996; 275: 1233 – 40.

[19] Badre R, Guillerm R, Abran N, Bourdin M, Dumas C. Pollution atmospherique par la fumee de tabac. *Ann. Pharm. Francaises.* 1978 ; 36 : 443 – 52.

[20] Elliot LP, Rowe DR. Air quality during public gatherings. *J. Air Poll. Control. Association.* 1975; 25: 635 – 6.

[21] Chappel SB, Parker RJ. Smoking and carbon monoxide levels in enclosed public places in New Brunswick. *Can. J. Public Health.* 1977; 68: 159 – 61.

[22] Coburn RF, Forster RE, Kane PB. Considerations of the physiological variables that determine the blood carboxyhemoglobin concentration in man. *J. Clin. Invest.* 1965; 44: 1899 – 910.

[23] Godin G, Wright G, Shephard RJ. Urban exposure to carbon monoxide. *Arch. Environ. Health.* 1972; 25: 305 – 13.

[24] Fischer T, Weber A, Grandjan E. Luftverunreinigung durch tabakrauch in gaststatten. *Int. Arch. Occup. Environ. Health.* 1978; 41: 267 – 80.

[25] Galuskinova V. 3,4 Benzopyrene determination in the smoky atmosphere of social meeting rooms and restaurants. A contribution to the problem of the noxiousness of so-called passive smoking. *Neoplasma.* 1964; 11: 465 – 8.

[26] Harlos DP, Marbury M, Samet J, Spengler JD. Relating indoor NO levels to infant personal exposures. *Atmospheric Environ.* 1987; 21: 369 – 76.

[27] Lebowitz MD, Burrows B. Respiratory symptoms related to smoking habits of family adults. *Chest.* 1976; 69: 48 – 50.

[28] Muramatsu M, Umemura S, Okada T, Tomita H. Estimation of personal exposure to tobacco smoke with a newly developed nicotine personal monitor. *Environ. Res.* 1984; 35: 218 – 27.

[29] Perry J. Fasten your seatbelts : No smoking. *Br. Columbia Med. J.* 1973; 15: 304 – 5.

[30] Sebben J, Pimm P, Shephard RJ. Cigarette smoke in enclosed public facilities. *Arch. Environ. Health.* 1977; 32: 52 – 8.

[31] Quant FR, Nelson PA, Sem GJ. Experimental measurements of aerosol concentrations in offices. *Environ. Int.* 1982; 8: 223 – 7.

[32] Hinds WC, First MW. Concentrations of nicotine and tobacco smoke public places. *N. Engl. J. Med.* 1975; 292: 844 – 5.

[33] Leone A, Mori L, Bertanelli F, Fabiano P, Filippelli M. Passive smoking: its effect on cardiac performance. *Int. J. Cardiol.* 1991; 8: 247 – 52.

[34] Wald NJ, Hackshaw AK. Cigarette smoking: an epidemiological overview. *Br. Med. Bulletin.* 1996; 52: 3 – 11.

[35] Haskell WL. Primer in preventive cardiology. In Pearson TA, Criqui MH, Luepker RV, Oberman A, Winston M eds. American Heart Association, Dallas 1994; 173 – 87.

[36] National Center for Health Statistics. Health, United States,1995. *DHHS pub no (PHS)* 96 – 1232. US Government Printing Office; 1996.

[37] American Heart Association. *Heart and Stroke Facts: 1995 Statistical Supplement.* American Heart Association, Dallas TX 75231, 1994; 4596.

[38] Leone A. The heart: a target organ for cigarette smoking. *J. Smoking-Related Dis.* 1992; 3: 197 – 201.

[39] Glantz SA, Parmley WW. Passive smoking and heart disease: epidemiology, physiology and biochemistry. *Circulation.* 1991; 83: 1 – 12.

[40] Wells AJ. Passive smoking as a cause of heart disease. *J. Am. Coll. Cardiol.* 1994; 24: 546 – 54.

[41] Glantz SA, Parmley WW. Passive smoking and heart disease. *JAMA.* 1995; 273: 1047 – 53.

[42] Kritz H, Schmid P, Sinzinger H. Passive smoking and cardiovascular risk. *Arch. Intern. Med.* 1995; 155: 1942 – 8.

[43] Leone A. Relationship between cigarette smoking and other coronary risk factors in atherosclerosis: risk of cardiovascular disease and preventive measures. *Curr. Pharm. Design.* 2003; 2417 – 23.

[44] Cook DG, Strachan DP. Health effects of passive smoking. Parental smoking and prevalence of respiratory symptoms and asthma in school age children. *Thorax.* 1997; 52: 1081 – 94.

[45] Hilton A. Stopping smoking: the importance of nicotine addiction. *Thorax.* 2000; 55: 256 – 7.

[46] Murray A, Morrison B. Passive smoking by asthmatics: its greater effect on boys than on girls and on older than on younger children. *Paediatrics.* 1989; 84: 451 – 9.

[47] Strachan DP, Cook DG. Health effects of passive smoking. Parenteral smoking and childhood asthma longitudinal and case-control studies. *Thorax.* 1998; 53: 204 – 12.

[48] Holt PG. Immune and inflammatory function in cigarette smokers. *Thorax.* 1987; 42: 241 – 9.

[49] Lee PN, Chamberlain J, Alderson MR. Relationship of passive smoking to risk of lung cancer and other smoking associated diseases. *Br. J. Cancer.* 1986; 54: 97 – 105.

[50] Hole DJ, Gillis CR, Chopra C, Hawthorne VM. Passive smoking and cardiorespiratory health in a general population in the west of Scotland. *Br. Med. J.* 1989; 299: 423 – 7.

[51] Hirayama T. Non-smoking wives of heavy smokers have a higher risk of lung cancer: a study from Japan. *Br. Med. J.* 1981; 282: 183 – 5.

[52] Kalandidi A, Trichopoulos D, Hatzakis A, Tzannes S, Saracci R. Passive smoking and chronic obstructive lung disease. *Lancet.* 1987; ii: 1325 – 6.

[53] Kauffmann F, Dockery DW, Speizer FE, Ferris BG. Respiratory symptoms and lung function in relation to passive smoking: a comparative study of American and French women. *Int. J. Epidemiol.* 1989; 18: 334 – 44.

[54] Masi MA, Hanley JA, Ernst P, Becklake MR. Environmental exposure to tobacco smoke and lung function in young adults. *Am. Rev. Respir. Dis.* 1988; 138: 296 – 9.

[55] Svendsen KH, Kuller LH, Martin MJ, Ockene JK. Effects of passive smoking in the multiple risk factor intervention trial. *Am. J. Epidemiol.* 1987; 126: 783 – 95.

[56] Hecht SS, Carmella SG, Murphy SE, Akerkar S, Brunnemann KD, Hoffmann D. A tobacco-specific lung carcinogen in the urine of men exposed to cigarette smoke. *N. Engl. J. Med.* 1993; 329: 1543 – 6.

[57] Nordenberg D, Yip R, Binkin NJ. The effect of cigarette smoking on hemoglobin levels and anemia screening. *JAMA*. 1990; 264: 1556 – 9.

[58] Bjork J, Albin M, Mauritzson N, Stromberg U, Johanson B, Hagmar L. Smoking and myelodysplastic syndromes. *Epidemiology*. 2000; 11: 285 – 91.

[59] Brownson RC. Cigarette smoking and risk of leukemia. *J. Clin. Epidemiol.* 1989; 42: 1025 – 6.

[60] Friedman GD. Cigarette smoking, leukemia, and multiple myeloma. *Ann. Epidemiol.* 1993; 3: 425 – 8.

[61] Pogoda JM, Preston-Martin S, Nichols PW, Ross RK. Smoking and risk of acute myeloid leukemia: results from a Los Angeles County case-control study. *Am. J. Epidemiol.* 2002; 155:546 – 53.

[62] Bain BJ. Does cigarette smoking cause leukaemia? *J. Smoking-Related Dis.* 1994; 5: 115 – 21.

[63] Garfinkel L. Time trends in lung cancer mortality among nonsmokers and a note on passive smoking. *J. Natl. Cancer Inst.* 1981; 66: 1061 – 6.

[64] Trichopoulos D, Kalandidi A, Sparros L. Lung cancer and passive smoking: conclusion of the Greek Study. *Lancet.* 1983; ii: 677 – 8.

[65] Hirayama T. Cancer mortality in nonsmoking women with smoking husbands based on a large-scale cohort study in Japan. *Prev. Med.* 1984; 13: 680 – 90.

[66] Garfinkel L, Auerbach O, Joubert L. Involuntary smoking and lung cancer: a case-control study. *J. Natl. Cancer Inst.* 1985; 75: 463 – 9.

[67] Humble CG, Samet JM, Pathak DR. Marriage to a smoker and lung cancer risk. *Am. J. Publ. Health.* 1987; 77: 5989 – 602.

[68] Wald NJ, Nanchahal K, Thompson SG, Cuckle HS. Does breathing other people's tobacco smoke cause lung cancer? *Br Med J* 1986; 293: 1217 – 22.

[69] Garland C, Barret-Connor E, Suarez L, Criqui MH, Wingard DL. Effects of passive smoking on ischemic heart disease mortality of nonsmokers. *Am J Epidemiol* 1985; 121: 645 – 50.

[70] Dobson AJ, Alexander HM, Heller RF, Lloyd DM. Passive smoking and the risk of heart attack or coronary death. *Med. J. Aust.* 1991; 154: 793 – 7.

[71] La Vecchia C, D'Avanzo B, Franzosi MG, Tognoni G. Passive smoking and the risk of acute myocardial infarction. *Lancet.* 1993; 341: 505 – 6.

[72] Correa P, Pickle LW, Fontham E, Lin Y, Haenszel W. Passive smoking and lung cancer. *Lancet.* 1983; ii: 595 – 7.

[73] Law MR, Hackshaw AK. Environmental tobacco smoke. *Br. Med. Bulletin.* 1996; 52: 22 – 34.

[74] He Y, Lam TH, Li LS, Li LS, Du RY, Jia GL, Huang JY, Zheng JS. Extent of coronary artery disease is associated with amount of passive smoking exposure. In *Tobacco and Health,* K Slama ed, Plenum Press, New York, 1995; 541 – 3.

[75] Leone A, Bertanelli F, Mori L, Fabiano P, Bertoncini G. Ventricular arrhythmias by passive smoke in patients with pre-existing myocardial infarction. *J. Am. Coll. Cardiol.* 1992; 3: 256A.

[76] Raitakari OT, Adams MR, McCredie RJ, Griffiths KA, Celermajer DS. Passive-smoke related arterial endothelial dysfunction is potentially reversible in healthy young adults. *Ann. Intern. Med.* 1999; 130: 578 – 81.

[77] Davis JW, Shelton L, Watanabe IS, Arnold J. Passive smoking affects endothelium and platelets. *Arch. Intern. Med.* 1989; 149: 386 – 9.

[78] Giannini D, Leone A, Nuti M, Strata G, Balbarini A, Mariani M. Indoor passive smoking impairs endothelial function. *European Heart J.* 2001; 22: 128A.

[79] Lough J. Cardiomyopathy produced by cigarette smoke. *Arch. Pathol. Lab. Med.* 1978; 102: 377 – 80.

[80] Celermajer DS, Sorensen KE, Georgakopoulos D. Cigarette smoking is associated with dose-related and potentially reversible impairment of endothelium-dependent dilation in healthy young adults. *Circulation.* 1993; 88: 2149 – 55.

[81] Kjeldsen K, Thomsen HK, Astrup P. Effects of carbon monoxide on myocardium. Ultrastructural changes in rabbits after moderate, chronic exposure. *Circ. Res.* 1974; 34: 339 – 48.

[82] Stefanidis C, Vlachopoulos C, Tsiamis E. Unfavorable effects of passive smoking in aortic function in men. *Ann. Intern. Med.* 1998; 128: 426 – 34.

Chapter 2

BIOCHEMICAL MARKERS OF PASSIVE SMOKING

ABSTRACT

Growing evidence of damage from several biochemical constituents of environmental tobacco smoke exists and plays a significant role in the development, maintaining, and progression of heart and blood vessels.

Some of these markers may be dosed in blood samples, urine and saliva, providing data about smoking exposure and amount of cardiovascular damage.

Among the thousands of chemical compounds of environmental tobacco smoke, usually rom nicotine, cotinine, carbon monoxide and thiocyanate have been dosed time by time, although these measures could not be conducted on a large-scale sample. At athe present time, cotinine concentrations, particularly in urine but also in blood and/or saliva, are preferably measured since cotinine dosage in urine is of easier determination than that of other metabolites to assess smoking exposure. Also, carboxyhemoglobin levels may provide qualitative but not quantitative data, unless in experimental studies, to estimate either the degree of cardiovascular damage or the level and duration of exposure.

Some hematologic markers may also be assessed to estimate smoking exposure, although with results worthwhile to be evaluated with prudence. Increased white blood cells, platelet aggregation and adhesiveness, fibrinogen level, and changes in serum lipids characterize chronic and prolonged smoking exposure.

Finally, smoking biomarkers, usually structured with chemically open chains, can cause possible chemical reactions into the tissues and organs of the body that can potentiate the harmful effects of smoking compounds, triggering, usually, a hypoxic mechanism that is further increased by a direct action of passive smoke components on cardiovascular system.

Keywords: Smoking Biomarkers, Nicotine, Cotinine, Carbon Monoxide, Thiocyanate, Chemistry, Toxicity, Measuring Method, Gas Chromatography, HPLC, HPLC coupled with Mass Spctrophotometry, Spectrophotometry, RIA, ELISA.

As it can be deduced from the previous chapter concerning the main characteristics of passive smoking, the chemical and biological nature of environmental tobacco smoke depends on the type and form of the tobacco products, characteristics of burned tobacco, environmental spaces, health and lifestyle of exposed subjects.

Among the thousands of components of passive smoking, those which particularly lead to cardiovascular damage are nicotine and its metabolites, carbon monoxide and thiocyanate. All together, these chemicals can cause every type of cardiovascular alterations described as a consequence of passive smoking exposure, although each compound can attack primarily some structures rather than others. Functional responses of heart and blood vessels may differ according to the prevalence of action of a tobacco chemical than that of another compound.

This chapter sets to focus on chemistry and main properties of those tobacco compounds (nicotine, carbon monoxide, and thiocyanate) that usually have negative effects on the cardiovascular system, their metabolic characteristics, pharmacological effects, evidence of damage caused, biochemical significance as markers of exposure to environmental tobacco smoke – and then dosage in biologic liquids – as well as markers of cardiovascular damage.

NICOTINE AND ITS METABOLITES

Nicotine [1] is a natural alkaloid with a basic charge obtained from the dried leaves and stems of the Nicotiana tabacum and Nicotiana rustica of Solanaceae family, where this compound varies in concentration from 0.5 percent to 8 percent. Nicotine biosynthesis takes place in the roots, and accumulates into the leaves, the particular shape and composition of which, described in Chapter 1, is a basic factor for the harvest and extraction of the alkaloid. Each cigarette, depending on its preparation, may reach nicotine concentration from 1.5 mg to 2.5 mg.

Chemistry

The structural formula for nicotine, the chemical name of which is 3(1-Methyl-2-pyrrolidinyl)pyridine, is C10H14N2 with a molecular mass of 162.23 g/mol. Nicotine stoechiometry looks like Figure 2.1.

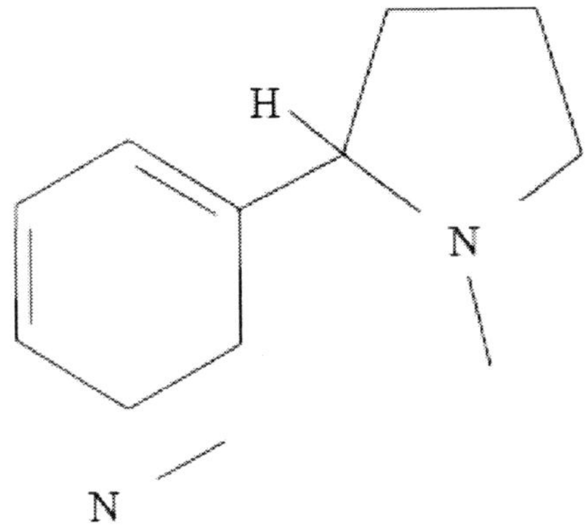

Figure 2.1. Chemical structure of nicotine.

Table 2.1. summarizes the main physico-chemical characteristics of the alkaloid.

Table 2.1. Physico-chemical characteristics of Nicotine

Chemical name	3-(1-Methyl-2-pyrrolidinyl)pyridine
Chemical nature	Alkaloid with a basic charge
Chemical formula	C10H14N2
Molecular mass	162.23 g/mol
Density	1.01 g/ml
Boiling point	247°C (degree of decomposition)
Melting point	-79°C
Autoignition temperature	240°C

Nicotine is a hygroscopic liquid that is miscible with water in its base form. Such a chemical characteristic makes the alkaloid diffusible on the whole tobacco leaf so that harvesting tobacco leaves fills up the greatest amount of nicotine. As a nitrogenous base, nicotine interacts with acid compounds forming salt that is usually soluble in water.

Assessing the physico-chemical properties of nicotine needs studies using different methodologies.

A study conducted using C14-labeled nicotine showed that about 15% of it was entering into the mainstream smoke, while as much as 37% characterized sidestream smoke with 18 % contained in the butt, and the remainder formed pyrolysis products [2]. As shown by Table 2.1, free base nicotine burns at a temperature of 240°C that is below its boiling point (247°C). Chemically, that means that nicotine is burned particularly when a cigarette is still smoked. The smoker then inhales the alkaloid, and the alkaloid also diffuses into the environment before its decomposition. Therefore, nicotine may almost entirely have adverse effects, the harmful of which is the addiction [3] that makes difficult to stop smoking. Although nicotine has the peculiar property of autoignition before its boiling point, a lower amount than the total of the tobacco leaf is dosable in the different types of smoke.

Pharmacodynamic and Metabolism

Absorption of nicotine by individuals occurs very quickly. Just in the oral cavity, there is an absorption that usually varies from 4% to 45% of the total dose [4]. However, as nicotine enters the body [5], it reaches the blood and then acts on those sites that are located at its specific receptors. Nicotinic acetylcholine receptors are those structures deputed to permit the biochemical action of the alkaloid.

These receptors feel the level of nicotine concentration. In the presence of small concentrations, the activity of the receptors arises whereas higher concentrations inhibit receptor activity. Such a condition explains the different responses of individuals to nicotine that can produce both stimulant and/or depressant effects. These effects are mediated through the interference with sympathetic system and then catecholamine levels. For the cardiovascular system, the heart, blood vessels, fat metabolism, carbohydrate metabolism, platelets and coagulation are particularly involved [6–14]. The main steps concerning the mechanisms through which nicotine causes cardiovascular changes are summarized in Figure 2.2.

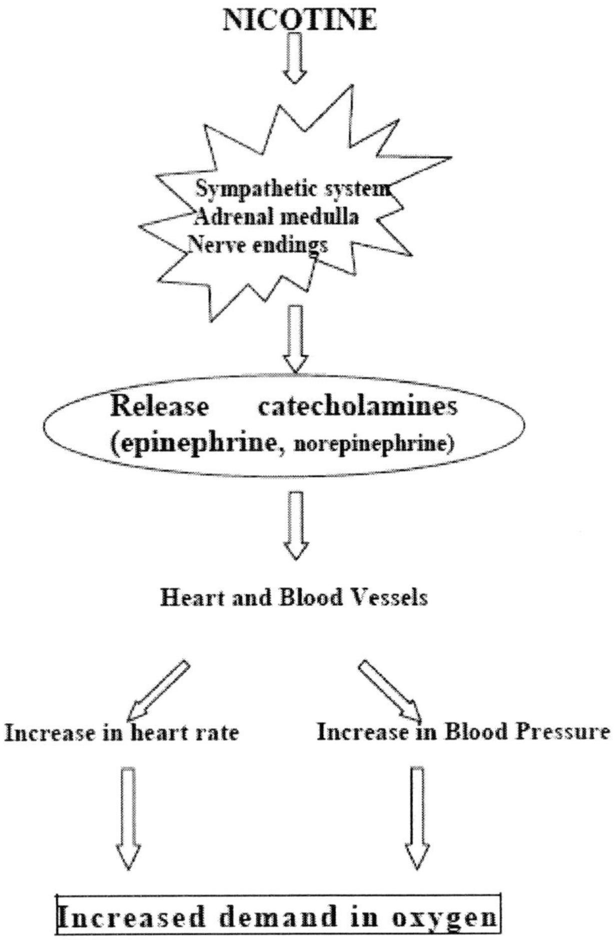

Figure 2.2. Mechanisms able to cause cardiovascular changes due to nicotine.

Nicotine exerts a direct and transiently repeated effect on sympathetic system and similar structures – chromaffin tissue - as well as the central nervous system. This effect is initially a stimulant effect, but it changes its characteristics and, in the long run, it becomes a depressant effect.

The exact mechanism by wich nicotine could trigger a cardiovascular event is yet to be completely clarified. However, a stimulation of sympathetic nerves and consequent release of intramyocardial catecholamines could be the primary cause [15–16].

Nicotine stimulates the release of norepinephrine from the hypotalamus and antidiuretic hormone from the pituitary gland [17]. Also chemoreceptors in the carotid artery can be stimulated by nicotine [18] triggering different reflexes.

Nicotine is metabolised to cotinine principally in the liver. The kidneys and lungs may be involved in the metabolism of the alkaloid, although with a little amount [19–20].

Table 2.2 lists nicotine pharmacodynamic.

Table 2.2. Nicotine pharmacodynamic

Absorption	Skin, oral mucosa, lungs
Transport	Blood component binding
Site of tissue binding	Nicotinic-acetylcholine receptors
Type of action	Sympathetic system effects
Metabolic steps	Liver (kidneys?, lungs?)
Main metabolite	Cotinine
Excretion	Urine

Carbon Monoxide

Carbon monoxide is a toxic gas not present in the fresh leaves of tobacco, but its formation about what is concerning cigarette smoke is due to decomposition into the burned cone of a cigarette by a chemical reaction with environmental oxygen and paper of the cigarette. Carbon monoxide present in the environment, produced by incomplete combustion of organic substances, comes from automobile exhausts, malfunctioning gas heaters, and tobacco smoke even if, in this case, at a smaller concentration than that of the two previous sources. However, the smaller environment concentrations of carbon monoxide could determine carboxyhemoglobin levels into the blood up to four times higher for nonsmokers exposed to passive smoking than those seen in similar populations not exposed [21]. Indeed, the bond between carbon monoxide and hemoglobin is about two hundred times stronger than that of oxygen and hemoglobin. Therefore, carbon monoxide can reduce oxyhemoglobin concentrations very easily with evident signs of hypoxia that affects different organs of the body, particularly cardiovascular system and brain.

Chemistry

Carbon monoxide is a colorless, odorless, tasteless gas which because of these properties and high toxicity is to be considered a potentially silent killer. Such a property is the result of the concentration level reached into the blood. Low concentrations act as a toxic factor, whereas the highest concentations lead rapidly to death.

The chemical formula for carbon monoxide is CO, a diatomic molecula with a bond between the two atoms carbon and oxygen as follows:

$$C = O$$

This type of bond is a basic characteristic for the chemical activity of carbon monoxide since it permits an easy dissociation in carbon atoms and oxygen atoms as well as an easy new linking with those substances towards which a major chemical affinity exists like blood hemoglobin. Usually, carbon monoxide is less dense than air and therefore, it is capable to spread out more quickly. It is also slightly soluble in water and burns in air, producing carbon dioxide.

The chemical characteristics of carbon monoxide are summarized in Table 2.3.

Table 2.3. Chemical characteristics of carbon monoxide

Chemical name	Carbon monoxide
Molecular formula	CO
Molar mass	28.01 g/mol
Physical characteristic	Colorless, Odorless gas
Solubility	Water, ethanol, methanol
Melting point	-205°C
Boiling point	-192°C
Structure	Linear molecular shape

Carbon monoxide is produced spontaneously into the body by a reaction between heme, a chemical component of hemoglobin, and an enzyme called heme-oxygenase in concentrations which are not a hazard for life.

Toxicity

Carbon monoxide is a very dangerous gas that may be fatal at a concentration as equal as 400 parts per million air.

Carbon monoxide toxicity due to cigarette smoking as well as passive smoking is the result of some complex reactions that are summarized in the Table 2.4.

Table 2.4. Steps of carbon monoxide toxicity from passive smoking

Step 1	Removing oxygen from oxyhemoglobin
Step 2	Replacement of oxygen with carbon monoxide
Step 3	Tissue hypoxia
Step 4	Impairment of cell metabolism

The mechanisms of damage consist of 4 phases: oxygen removing and its replacement with carbon monoxide, formation of carboxyhemoglobin —these first two steps of removing and replacement have to be keep in mind with care since they are the chemical factors which trigger the toxic action of carbon monoxide from passive smoking exposure—, tissue hypoxia, and then impairment of cellular metabolism. Furthermore, carbon monoxide plays its action directly, even if at lower concentrations, on intracellular structures inhibiting respiratory metabolism of the cells and intracellular constituents [22–30], particularly those RNA-related.

The percentage of carboxyhemoglobin in the body determines the type of symptoms and level of damage that may be experienced.

Finally, fatal effects due to acute exposure to relatively high concentrations of carbon monoxide, are the result of a direct action of the gas on cardiorespiratory and nervous structures of the body with consequent fatal respiratory and cardiac arrest preceded by irreversible coma.

THIOCYANATE

Thiocyanate [1] is a chemical substance widely distributed in nature, and occuring in biological liquids such as blood, saliva, and urine. Many plants, particularly of the genus Brassica (cabbages) contain this product. Thiocyanate interferes with different steps of body metabolism [31–34], particularly with iodine metabolism [32], and causes levels of tissue alterations that can vary with regard to types of food consumed, characteristics of living environment, health of the subjects, and possible presence of previous diseases particularly affecting the thyroid gland.

Thiocyanate is present in the vapor phase of tobacco smoke usually in the form of hydrogen cyanide. Industrially, it is used in agriculture to prepare insecticides and fungicides, in car industries as a fuel for airbags, and in pharmaceutical industries to prepare antibiotics, thyroid drugs, and chemotherapic drugs. The effects of this substance on cardiovascular system particularly after chronic exposure to passive smoking are added to those of nicotine and carbon monoxide with potentiating their toxicity. Isolatedly it is very difficult to identify the effects of thiocyanate alone from passive smoking on cardiovascular system.

Chemistry

Thiocyanate is a colourless, odorless crystalline powder with a chemical formula that changes according to the type of salt linked to thiocyanate structure that is: – SCN -. Among the different salts, potassium and sodium are more frequently used to constitute the molecular formula that is KSCN for potassium salt and NaSCN for sodium salt.

Spatially, thiocyanate is structured as follows:

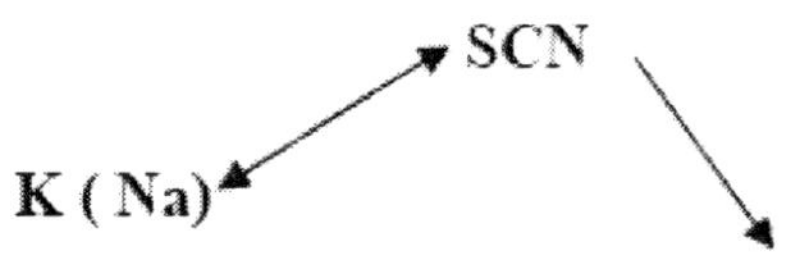

The chemical characteristics of thiocyanate are listed in table 2.5.

Table 2.5. Chemical characteristics of thiocyanate

Appearance	Colourless, odorless crystal
Solubility	Water (very soluble)
Density	1.89
Boiling point	500°C
Melting point	173°C
Stability	Slow decomposition under light
Decomposition products	Nitrogen oxides, solfur compounds

Toxicity

Hydrogen cyanide is metabolized in the liver with production of thiocyanate by a series of chemical reactions that involve enzymatic chains, organic substrates, and shift of metabolic steps. Cyanide is acutely toxic to humans. However, the amount of cyanide inhaled following exposure to passive smoking usually determines symptoms of chronic intoxication or more frequently potentiates the harmful effects on cardiovascular system due to nicotine and carbon monoxide, as aforesaid.

The toxicity of hydrogen cyanide depends particularly from the nature of the exposure. The time, dose and manner of exposure are the main parameters to be evaluated to assess the degree of toxicity. However, when cyanide enters the blood, it forms a stable complex with a particular form of cytochrome oxidase, an enzyme usually deputed to permit the synthesis of ATP. The reduced amount of cytochrome oxidase causes a decrease in ATP synthesis with consequently troubles in mitochondria structure and metabolism, shift of aerobic to anaerobic metabolism, and accumulation of lactate into the blood. The concomitant hypoxia due to carbon monoxide of environmental tobacco smoke potentiates the negative effects of cyanide on the cardiovascular system. Figure 2.3. schematizes the main steps of cyanide metabolism.

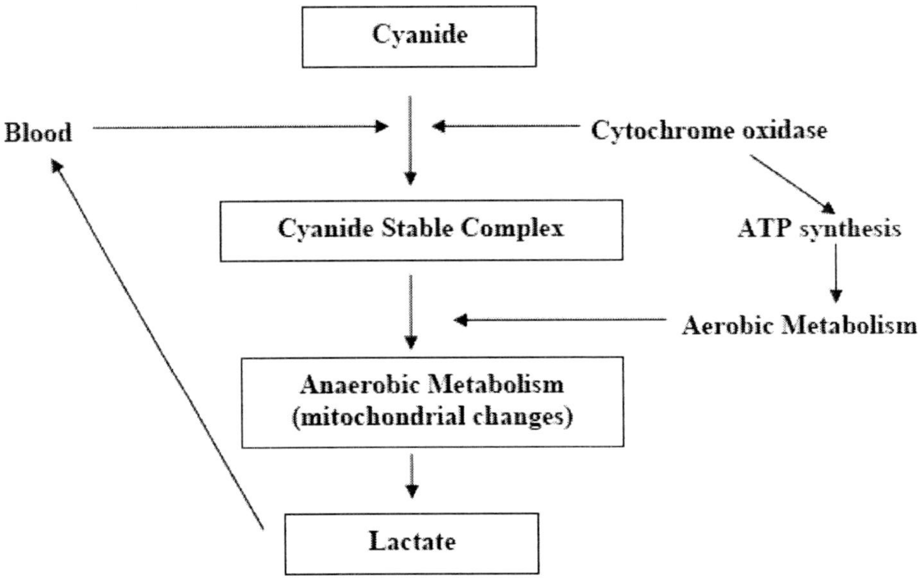

Figure 2.3. The main steps of cyanide metabolism into the body.

Cyanide is converted into the body to thiocyanate, which interacts with thiosulfates by a chemical reaction catalyzed by sulfur transferase enzymes. Thiocyanate is the compound that can be dosed, although with difficulty, because of its excretion in the urines. However, the metabolic steps that lead to formation of thiocyanate from hydrogen cyanide produce a chemical compound that is about seven times less toxic than that of the original substance.

Symptoms of cyanide poisoning usually occur from an exposure of 20 to 40 ppm of cyanide vapor phase, a concentration very difficult to reach in both acute or chronic passive smoking exposure. Headache, drowsiness, vertigo, confusion, and changes in pulse and breathing that become deeper and more rapid are the initial symptoms of cyanide intoxication (Table 2.6). These symptoms are followed, in case of higher cyanide concentrations or more prolonged exposure, by convulsions, dilated pupils, and clammy skin. A third phase of intoxication is characterized by pulse rate and irregular breathing with a fall of body temperature, resulting in, coma, heart and breath arrest followed by death.

Table 2.6. Symptoms of cyanide intoxication

Phase 1.	Headache, vertigo, drowsiness, rapid pulse, rapid and deep breathing, nausea, vomiting.
Phase 2.	Convulsions, dilated pupils, clammy skin.
Phase 3.	Pulse rate and breathing widely irregular, fall in body temperature
Phase 4.	Coma, cardiorespiratory arrest, death.

These phases that characterize cyanide intoxication are absolutely inexistent in the presence of passive smoking. However, this knowledge helps to keep in mind the harmful effects of cyanide and its metabolites.

Main characteristic of cyanide compounds, similarly to what occurs for the nicotine in passive smoking but not for carbon monoxide, is the rapidity to produce human body metabolites usually less toxic than the original substances and also dosable to assess passive smoking exposure. For cyanide, the salts of sodium and/or potassium particularly note such a condition.

PASSIVE SMOKING CHEMICALS AS BIOMARKERS

Cardiovascular alterations due to smoking exposure can be identified by assessing some biochemical markers that are currently used either as diagnostic markers of smoking exposure or markers that allows the evaluation and/or follow the course of some specific lesions of the heart and blood vessels.

Nicotine and its metabolites [35], carbon monoxide and serum thiocyanate [36] are the most widely used biomarkers of smoking exposure, although their biochemical assessing can undergo difficult dosage.

Different methods are used to quantify smoking products, and also differences in each method with regard to the type of chemical substance to be dosed. Table 2.7 lists the most frequently used methods for the assessment of tobacco smoke compounds. All these methods measure particularly cotinine [20, 35, 36–44], the main metabolite of nicotine. Its measure may provide useful data about smoking habit, type of exposure to environmental smoke, and frequency of exposure. Moreover, the costs borne to assess the concentrations of cotinine are much less expensive than those due to dosing the other smoking compounds, and also easier to be performed in a large majority of cases, unless carboxyhemoglobin is in the blood,.

Table 2.7. Methods most frequently used for assessing tobacco smoke compounds

Method	Chemical compound
Gas Chromatography	Cotinine, Nicotine
HPLC	Cotinine, Nicotine
HPLC coupled with mass spectrophotometry	Cotinine, Nicotine, Caffeine
RIA	Cotinine
ELISA	Cotinine
Fluorescence Polarization Immunoassay	Cotinine

Examining Table 2.7, there is evidence that methods used to assess the markers of smoking exposure can be classified into three groups: physical methods, immunological methods, and radioimmunoassay methods. All these methods are a good indicator of both active and passive smoking exposure in epidemiological surveys [45–46]. However, methods cannot be used in a large-scale epidemiological trials because they need particularly specialised laboratories.

Gas Chromatography

Generally, chromatography is a physico-chemical method that utilizes the separation of chemically mixed compounds into separate components. By performing this procedure, a sample is decomposed to its individual substances making this separation easier to identify either qualitatively or quantitatively, and then measurable in amount of the different sample components.

Among the different chromatographic techniques, gas chromatography is widely used, allowing the analysis of up to 20 percent of chemical compounds. However, undergoing gas chromatographic analysis, a compound must have at least two specific properties: sufficient volatility and thermal stability. Smoking compounds in vapor phase have these characteristics [39].

In gas chromatography technique, a chemical sample in vapor-phase is injected onto chromatographic columns and then separated into its components by an elution process due to the flow of an inert gas, usually helion, argon or nitrogen, that functions as mobile phase without any molecular interaction with the components of the analyzed mixture. The mobile phase moves the eluted components of the mixture that are then immobilized from a column containing a solid gas – stationary phase – that absorbs each individual component at a level depending on its chemical bonding and concentration. By doing so, each substance is separated from the other components of the mixture and then assessed qualitatively and quantitatively.

Among the different toxic chemicals of environmental tobacco smoke, particularly nicotine and cotinine can be dosed by gas chromatographic technique [39, 47].

HPLC and HPLC Coupled with Mass Spectrophotometry

The method HPLC, namely High Pressure Liquid Cromatography, is a good predictor, similarly to the other methods listed in this section, of cotinine and nicotine concentrations in biological liquids of both active smokers and nonsmokers chronically exposed to environmental tobacco [40–41].

It determines a separation of one chemical substance from another utilizing their absorption of ultraviolet light as well as the interaction of the compound to be dosed with an analytical column substrate, an essential structure of the system, equipped with different chemistries according to the nature of the chemical to be determined.

An HPLC system consists of the following instruments, all used for a correct assessment of the chemical substance to measure:

1. A pump (solvent delivery system);
2. An automatic Injector;
3. A column with different chemistries;
4. An UV Detector (different detectors such as fluorescent detector, conductivity dectector etc. All these detectors give results that are clearly not better than those obtained by using an UV detector);
5. An Analytical Data System that may be a computer or a common recorder.

These instruments are typically small so that they can be placed usefully in specialised laboratories.

HPLC is often used associated with a mass spectrophotometry instrument for a more sensitive analysis of urinary cotinine and caffeine [41] concentrations in an attempt to better establish smoking exposure.

RIA

RIA is the abbreviation of Radioimmunoassay. This method [48] utilizes the principle based on the property that a fixed concentration of a labeled tracer antigen is incubated with an antiserum at a known concentration, so that the binding sites of antigen with an antibody are occupied only for a limited portion. Therefore, there are sites of the labeled tracer antigen that are free from any binding. When an unlabeled antigen is added to this complex, a competition between labeled tracer and unlabeled antigen exists, particularly for the limited and constant number of binding sites on the antibody. Therefore, the amount of tracer bound to the antibody will decrease progressively when concentrations of the unlabeled antigen increase. Then, measuring can be performed after separating antibody-bound from free tracer and determining either the bound fraction, the free fraction or both components. A calibration of the system needs to measure the amount of the different fractions and a standard curve is then set up with increasing levels of known antigen, and from this curve the amount of antigen in unknown samples will be calculated.

Basic factors in a radioimmunoassay system are:

1. an antiserum of the compound to be measured;
2. the availability of a radioactively labeled form of the compound;
3. a system whereby antibody-bound tracer can be separated from the amount of unbound tracer;
4. those standard unlabeled materials that need to perform RIA.

Nicotine and particularly cotinine can be assessed carefully by using RIA method [42], although these dosages also require specialized laboratories.

ELISA

ELISA, Enzyme-Linked ImmunoSorbant Assay, is a method [49] directed towards measuring a particular protein when it enters into a sample and if so, how its concentration occurs. This method utilizes both an antibody and enzyme reactions, and the amount of compound to be dosed will be assessed by using a system of optical density that analyzes the amount of color produced. The amount of color produced is proportional to the amount of substance present in the analyzed sample.

Two main variations characterize this method. A first method is to determine how much antibody is in a sample, while a second method determines how much protein is bound by an antibody. The first case permits to better quantify an antibody; in the second case, the attention is directed towards the proteins.

ELISA is a widely used method to assess biological markers in different fields of the medicine. For what is concerning tobacco smoke exposure, cotinine in saliva and urine of active and passive smokers would seem to provide effective data [43].

Nicotine and cotinine are the biomarkers most widely dosed with the current methods of analysis, although their determination requires specialized laboratories. Moreover, cotinine, a major metabolite of nicotine, is used more widely as a smoking biomarker since its urinary concentration has been considered one of the most specific and representative parameter for tobacco smoke exposure [20, 35, 37–38, 50].

Urinary cotinine values are significantly higher in nonsmokers after their exposure to environmental smoke. Such a fact has been well documented in children [47] exposed to environmental tobacco smoke if they were compared to non-exposed children. Indeed, urinary cotinine concentrations were statistically higher in those children exposed with a statistical significance of a great degree (a "P" value less than 0.001 was calculated, while a value limit statistically significant is 0.05).

In a large study that enrolled pregnant women [51], cotinine concentrations were higher in non smoking women who were passively exposed to cigarette smoke than in those who were not exposed, and urinary cotinine levels further increased in the cases of more prolonged exposure to environmental tobacco smoke. Finally, cotinine levels in those women who smoked were higher after childbirth than during pregnancy.

In conclusion, nicotine and cotinine may affect cardiovascular system similarly, although the harmful effects of nicotine can be seen preferably after acute exposure to tobacco smoke [50], being earlier than those due to cotinine. The last metabolite acts longer and it is biochemically better determined in study samples.

Carbon Monoxide

Biological monitoring of carbon monoxide inhalation from cigarette combustion and passive smoking exposure may be desumed by the dosage of carboxyhemoglobin. But, the exact assessment of how much increased carboxyhemoglobin levels are due to passive smoking exposure often fails because of the large presence of carbon monoxide as a pollutant in different environmental sites such as industries, car fuel and others. There should be carboxyhemoglobin levels before passive smoking exposure and then after smoking exposure to determine the effective amount of this substance due to environmental tobacco smoke. That is particularly possible under experimental procedures [21] that provide for carboxyhemoglobin measure before and then after acute smoking exposure.

However, carboxyhemoglobin can be satisfactory dosed in an arterial blood sample or, more easily, in a venous blood sample, which must be collected in a closed container containing an anticoagulant of the type dry sodium heparine or disodium ethylene-diaminotetracetic acid (EDTA). Then, blood samples must be preserved, also for several days, prior to analysis but they must be kept cold (4°C) and in the dark and then measured by spectrophotometric methods [52–55].

Another useful approach to estimate the exposure to carbon monoxide [21] is the analysis of the gas in the expired air after smoking exposure. The percent difference between the amount of gas expired after exposure and that expired before provides data concerning the course of the phenomenon.

In conclusion, the importance of carbon monoxide as a biomarker of passive smoking exposure is worthy of being considered on condition that pre-exposure levels of carboxyhemoglobin are known and the amount of environmental pollutants containing this gas are not produced by the estimated smoking.

Usually, the amount of carboxyhemoglobin following acute exposure to passive smoking at a concentration 30 – 35 ppm of the gas may increase from twice to four times the values [21] detected before exposure.

Thiocyanate

Cigarette smoking commonly releases this chemical that is present in smoking vapor phase as hydrogen cyanide. Both active smokers and non smokers exposed to environmental tobacco smoke have a mean blood thiocyanate levels of about 0.4 mcg/ml. These levels are from two to two and a half times greater than the levels of persons who do not smoke or are not exposed to smoking products. Usually, these people have a normally mean thiocyanate blood concentrations of about 0.15 to 0.20 mcg/ml.

Thiocyanate in serum [31–34] has been monitored preferably in the past particularly to assess the effectiveness of cigarette smoking cessation programs and also in experimental animal studies [56]. This monitoring has been rapidly replaced by the measurement of cotinine or nicotine levels in serum and urine for practical reasons: easier dosage of the last chemicals, and lack of interference with some foods which could and can, otherwise, influence thiocyanate metabolism. Milk, almonds, garlic, onion, leek, cabbage and cauliflower contribute to a mild elevation in serum thiocyanate concentrations. Such an occurence may make it difficult to separate nonsmokers from smokers or nonsmokers exposed to passive smoke as well as to establish the behaviour of smokers in smoking cessation programs.

Several other biomarkers have been, from time to time, proposed as potential toxics which permit to assess either smoking exposure or cardiovascular damage [57]: anabasine, anatabine, benzene, hydroxypyrene, aromatic compounds. However, they have been rapidly left since there were evident difficulties for their dosage and, at the same time, their assessment did not provide clearer results than those obtained by dosing nicotine and, particularly, cotinine.

Hematologic Biochemical Markers

An interesting factor to underline is the behavior of some hematologic markers which may be influenced and often changed by chronic passive smoking exposure [58–62]. These markers may be easily investigated by a routine hematologic examination, although they are not specific markers of smoking exposure and if they are changed from tobacco smoke, the exposure, particularly in the case of passive exposure, must last for a long time that may be calculated in several years. However, when these parameters change for passive smoking exposure, there is a real clinical problem either to lead back their values or remove those biochemical and structural alterations which maintain their change.

The main parameters, which can be influenced by environmental smoke exposure, are listed in Table 2.8. Some parameters increase their activity or blood concentrations as an effect of passive smoking exposure, whereas some others undergo reduced blood concentrations. Moreover, some of these parameters change more quickly and transiently being related also to the cardiovascular response of acute exposure.

Table 2.8. Hematologic parameters mainly related to smoking exposure

Platelet changes (increased aggregation and adhesiveness)
Increased plasma catecholamines
Increased LDL-Cholesterol
Increased fibrinogen level
Increased Factor VII
Increased Plasma viscosity
Increased leukocyte count
Increased reactive C protein
Decreased Plasminogen
Decreased serum estrogens

In conclusion, smoking habit may be carefully determined by the dosage of cotinine in urine, blood and saliva more than that of other markers. However, for nicotine and cotinine, there are yet limits evident on their large-scale use. Blood, urine, and saliva are the samples usually used to dose cotinine and thiocyanate; blood and urine samples are used for measuring nicotine concentrations; at least, carbon monoxide may be dosed in both blood and expired air.

These biochemical markers due to environmental tobacco smoke exposure have harmful effects on heart and blood vessels usually after prolonged chronic exposure of individuals, unless some experimental cases in which, acute exposure was studied at standard concentrations [7, 21, 63– 64].

These biomarkers, which are chemically structured with open terminal chains, can determine chemical reactions with the components of different tissues and organs of the body with production of other chemicals, often less toxic than the original compounds but sometimes more harmful, which can potentiate the negative effects due to environmental tobacco smoke. Such a fact could be carefully considered with regard to the possibility of these interferences. However, in the large majority of cases, a hypoxic mechanism with consequent metabolic and structural damage triggers those alterations usually attributed to passive smoking exposure and that will be described in more detail the later chapters.

There is evidence that hypoxia damages heavily different structures of the body, particularly in older persons and in those persons who are suffering from previous ischemic events. Structural alterations of myocardium due to direct action of carbon monoxide on cardiovascular system have also been seen [27, 29 –30, 65].

These two factors, hypoxia and directly damaging action on cardiovascular system , determined by environmental tobacco smoke compounds, usually maintain the degree of cardiovascular damage giving it, in the long run, a characteristic of irreversibility.

Until a breakdown, there is a linear relationship between the levels of biochemical markers and level of cardiovascular alterations, in the sense that the occurence of an irreversible lesion usually frees from the measures of biochemical markers, that could also be reduced, avoiding smoking exposure, and maintaining and making progress according to the type of cardiovascular damage. Therefore, the evidence of an hypoxic damage in individuals who had been previously exposed to environmental tobacco smoke and later stopped the exposure, could be a consequence of prolonged exposure, even if hematologic or urinary biochemical markers of smoking exposure provide normal concentrations.

A clear example of that is given by the effects of nicotine and carbon monoxide on blood pressure. Some reports [66] concerning the relationship between cigarette smoking and blood pressure emphasize tobacco smoke as a factor able to induce hypotension, whereas other reports [67–68] underline that hypertension is the late result of smoking exposure. There is, therefore, an evident disagreement that could be explained as follows. After a temporary increase in blood pressure levels due to vasoconstriction for enhanced catecholamine release mediated by nicotine [6, 16-19] and autonomic system stimulation, the depressant effects of this metabolite cause vasodilation, which is responsible for lower blood pressure levels. At the same time, the heart and blood vessels are damaged because of a direct action of carbon monoxide and in time the alterations caused by this gas become irreversible. Therefore, blood pressure tends to reach higher levels again as a consequence of irreversibly pathological lesions. Thus, hypertension usually affects eldery people who smoke cigarettes or are exposed to tobacco products for a longer time.

Finally, the results obtained by the studies on the relationship between smoking and blood pressure provide the evidence of an interaction among the different biochemical markers of smoking that can lead to masking, at the beginning and cardiovascular damage that will be clearly evident when irreversible alterations can be seen.

REFERENCES

[1] Kice JL, Marvell EN. *Modern Principles of Organic Chemistry. An Introduction.* 3rd ed, The Macmillan Company, New York, USA, 1967.

[2] Houseman TH. Studies of cigarette smoke transfer using radioisotopically labelled tobacco constituents. Part II. The transference of radioisotopically labelled nicotine to cigarette smoke. *Beitrage zur Tabakforschung.* 1973; 7: 142 – 7.

[3] US Department of Health and Human Services. *The health consequences of smoking: Nicotine addiction.* Washington DC, US Government Printing Office; 1988.

[4] Armitage AK, Turner DM. Absorption of nicotine in cigarette and cigar smoke through the oral mucosa. *Nature.* 1970; 226: 1231 – 2.

[5] Armitage AK, Dollery CT, George CF, Houseman TH, Lewis PJ, Turner DM. Absorption and metabolism of nicotine from cigarettes. *Br. Med. J.* 1975; 4: 313 – 6.

[6] Leone A. Cigarette smoking and health of the heart. *J. Roy. Soc. Health.* 1995; 115: 354 – 5.

[7] Aronow WS. Effect of passive smoking on angina pectoris. *N. Engl. J. Med.* 1978; 299: 21 – 4.

[8] Glantz SA, Parmley WW. Passive smoking and heart disease : epidemiology, physiology, and biochemistry. *Circulation.* 1991; 83: 1 – 12.

[9] Celermejer DS, Sorensen KE, Georgakopoulos D. Cigarette smoking is associated with dose-related and potentially reversible impairment of endothelium-dependent dilation in healthy young adults. *Circulation.* 1993; 88: 2149 – 55.

[10] Leone A. Relationship between cigarette smoking and other coronary risk factors in atherosclerosis : risk of cardiovascular disease and preventive measures. *Curr. Pharm. Design.* 2003; 9: 2417 – 23.

[11] Glantz SA, Parmley WW. Passive smoking and heart disease. *JAMA.* 1995; 273: 1047 – 53.

[12] Leone A, Giannini D, Bellotto C, Balbarini A. Passive smoking and coronary heart disease. *Current Vascular Pharmacology.* 2004; 2: 175 – 82.

[13] Fielding JE, Phenow KJ. Health effects of involuntary smoking. *N. Engl. J. Med.* 1988; 319: 1452 – 60.

[14] Powell JT. Vascular damage from smoking: disease mechanisms at the arterial wall. *Vasc. Med.* 1998; 3: 21 – 8.

[15] Ball K, Turner R. Smoking and the heart: the basis for action. *Lancet.* 1974; 2: 822 – 6.

[16] Benowitz NL, Jacob P III, Jones RT, Rosemberg J. Interindividual variability in the metabolism and cardiovascular effects of nicotine in man. *Journal of Pharmacology and Experimental Therapeutics.* 1982; 221: 368 – 72.

[17] Castro de Souza EM, Silva MRE Jr. The release of vasopressin by nicotine: Further studies on its site of action. *J. Physiol.* 1977; 265: 297 – 311.

[18] Cohen AJ, Roe FJC. Monograph on the Pharmacology and Toxicology of Nicotine. *Tobacco Advisory Council Occasional Paper.* 4, 1981; London, 45.

[19] Turner DM, Armitage AK, Briant RH, Dollery CT. Metabolism of nicotine by the isolated perfused dog lung. *Xenobiotica.* 1975; 5: 539 – 51.

[20] Benowitz NL. Cotinine as a biomarker of environmental tobacco smoke exposure. *Epidemiol. Rev.* 1996; 18: 188 – 204.

[21] Leone A, Mori L, Bertanelli F, Fabiano P, Filippelli M. Indoor passive smoking: its effect on cardiac performance. *Int. J. Cardiol.* 1991; 8: 247 – 52.

[22] Adams JD, Erickson HH, Stone HL. Myocardial metabolism during exposure carbon monoxide in the conscious dog. *J. appl. Physiol.* 1973; 34: 238 – 42

[23] Horwath SM, Raven PB, Dahms TE, Gray DJ. Maximal aerobic capacity at different levels of carboxyhemoglobin. *J. appl. Physiol.* 1975; 38: 300 – 3.

[24] Lewey FH, Drabkin DD. Experimental chronic carbon monoxide poisoning of dogs. *Am. J. Med. Sci.* 1944; 208: 502 – 11.

[25] Ehrich WE, Bellet S, Lewey FH. Cardiac changes from CO poisoning. *Am. J. Med. Sci.* 1944; 208: 512 – 23.

[26] Musselman NP, Groff WA, Yevich PP, Wilinsky FT, Weeks MH, Oberst FW. Continuous exposure of laboratory animals to low concentration of carbon monoxide. *Aerosp. Med.* 1959; 30: 524 – 9.

[27] Astrup P. Some physiological and pathological effects of moderate carbon monoxide exposure. *Br. Med. J.* 1972; 4: 447 – 52.

[28] Anderson RF, Allensworth DC, DeGroot WJ. Myocardial toxicity from carbon monoxide poisoning. *Ann. Int. Med.* 1967; 11:72 – 82.

[29] Kjeldsen K, Thomsen HK, Astrup P. Effects of carbon monoxide on myocardium. Ultrastructural changes in rabbits after moderate, chronic exposure. *Circ. Res.* 1974; 34: 339 – 48.

[30] Thomsen HK, Kjeldsen K. Threshold limit for carbon monoxide-induced myocardial damage. *Arch. Environ. Health.* 1974; 29: 73 – 8.

[31] Apple FS. Serum thiocyanate concentrations in patients with normal or impaired renal function receiving nitroprusside. *Clin. Chem.* 1996; 42: 1878 – 9.

[32] De la Higuera AJ. Determination of serum thiocyanate in patients with thyroid disease using a modification of the Aldridge method. *J. Anal. Toxicol.* 1994; 18: 58 – 9.

[33] Diagnostic Bulletin. Serum thiocyanate as a marker for exposure to tobacco smoke. *Lab. Report for Physicians.* 1985; 7: 63.

[34] Olea F, Parras P. Determination of serum levels of dietary thiocyanate. *J. Anal. Toxicol.* 1992; 16: 258 – 60.

[35] Benowitz NL, Jacob P. Nicotine and cotinine elimination pharmacokinetics in smokers and non smokers. *Clin. Pharmacol. Ter.* 1993; 53: 316 – 23.

[36] Vogt TM, Selvin S, Widdowson G, Hulley SB. Expired air carbon monoxide and serum thiocyanate as objective measures of cigarette exposure. *Am. J. Public Health.* 1977; 67: 545 – 9.

[37] Apselhoff G, Ashton HM, Friedman H, Gerber N. The importance of measuring cotinine levels to identify smokers in clinical trials. *Clin. Pharmacol. Ther.* 1994; 56:460 – 2.

[38] Jarvis MJ, Tunstall-Pedoe H, Feyerabend C, Vesey C, Saloojee Y. Comparison of tests used to distinguish smokers from non smokers. *Am. J. Public Health.* 1987; 77: 1435 – 8.

[39] Feyerabend C, Russel MAH. A rapid gas-liquid chromatographic method for the determination of cotinine and nicotine in biological fluids. *J. Pharm. Pharmacol.* 1999; 42: 450 – 2.

[40] James H, Tibazi Y, Taylor R. Rapid method for the simultaneous measurement of nicotine and cotinine in urine and serum by gas-chromatography-mass spectrometry. *J. Chromatogr. B.* 1998; 708: 87 – 93.

[41] Tuomi T, Johnson T, Reijula K. Analysis of nicotine, 3-hydroxycotinine, cotinine and caffeine in urine of passive smokers by HPLC-tandem mass spectrometry. *Clin. Chem.* 1999; 45: 2164 – 72.

[42] Langone JJ, Gjika HB, Van Vunakis H. *Nicotine and its metabolites.* Radioimmunoassay for nicotine and cotinine. i 1973; 12: 5025 – 30.

[43] Langone JJ, Cook G, Bjercke R, Lifshitz MH. Monoclonal antibody ELISA for cotinine in saliva and urine of active and passive smokers. *J. Immunol. Methods.* 1988; 114: 74 – 8.

[44] Ekemin SA, Coxon RE, Colbert DL, Landon J, Smith DS. Urinary cotinine fluoroimmunoassay for smoking status screening adapted to an automated analyser. *Analyst.* 1992; 117: 697 – 9.

[45] Greenberg RA, Haley NJ, Ersel RA, Loda FA. Measuring the exposure of infants to tobacco smoke. *N. Engl. J. Med.* 1984; 310: 1075 – 8.

[46] Strachan DP, Jarvis MJ, Feyerabend C. Passive smoking, salivary cotinine concentrations and middle ear effusion in 7-year-old children. *Br. Med. J.* 1989; 289: 1549 – 52.

[47] Roche D, Callais F, Reungoat P, Momas I. Adaptation of an enzyme immunoassay to assess urinary cotinine in nonsmokers exposed to tobacco smoke. *Clin. Chem.* 2001; 47: 950 –2.

[48] *Principles of the Radioimmunoassay- RIA Method* -, maintained by F Wegner, 2003 University of Wisconsin System Board of Reagents.

[49] ELISA. Department of Biology, Davidson College, Davidson, NC; 2002.

[50] Leone A. Biochemical markers of cardiovascular damage from tobacco smoke. *Curr. Pharm. Design.* 2005; 11: 2199 – 208.

[51] Spierto FW, Hannon WH, Kendrick JS, Bernert JT, Pirkle J, Gargiullo P. Urinary cotinine levels in women enrolled in a smoking cessation study during and after pregnancy. *J. Smoking-Related Dis.* 1994; 5: 65 – 76.

[52] Drabkin DL, Austin JH. Spectrophotometric studies. II. Preparation from washed blood cells; nitric oxide hemoglobin and sulfhemoglobin. *J. biol. Chem.* 1935; 112: 51 – 65.

[53] Malenfant AL, Gambino SR, Waraska AJ, Roe EL. Spectrophotometric determination of hemoglobin concentration and percent oxyhemoglobin and carboxyhemoglobin saturation. *Clin. Chem.* 1968; 14: 789.

[54] Small KA, Radford EP, FrazierJM, Rodkey FL, Collison HA. A rapid method for simultaneous measurement of carboxy and methemoglobin in blood. *J. appl. Physiol.* 1971; 31: 154 – 60

[55] Lily REC, Cole PV, Hawkins LH. Spectrophotometric measurements of carboxyhemoglobin. *Br. J. Ind. Med.* 1972; 29: 454 – 7.

[56] Rogers WR, Bass III RL, Johnson DE, Kruski AW, McMahan CA, Montiel MM, Mott GE, Wilbur RL, McGill HC Jr. Atherosclerosis-related responses to cigarette smoking in the baboon. *Circulation.* 1980; 61: 1188 – 93.

[57] Hatsukami DK, Hecht SS, Hennrikus DJ, Joseph AM, Pentel PR. Biomarkers of tobacco exposure or harm: Application to clinical and epidemiological studies. *Nicotine and Tobacco Research* 2003;5: 387 – 96.

[58] Muscat JE, Harris RE, Haley NY, Wynder EL. Cigarette smoking and plasma cholesterol. *Am. Heart J.* 1991; 121: 141 – 7.

[59] Imaizumi T, Satoh K, Yoshida H, Kawamura Y, Hiramoto M, Takamatsu S. Effect of cigarette smoking on the levels of platelet-activating factor-like lipid(s) in plasma lipoproteins. *Atherosclerosis.* 1991; 87: 47 – 55.

[60] Becker C, Dubin T. Activation of Factor XII by tobacco glycoprotein. *J. Exp. Med.* 1977; 146: 457 – 67.

[61] Saba S, Mason R. Some effects of nicotine on platelet. *Thromb. Res.* 1975; 7: 819 – 24.

[62] Ou X, Ramos K. Benzo(a)pyrene inhibits protein kinase C activity in subcultured rat aortic smooth muscle cells. *Chem. Biol. Interact.* 1994; 91: 29 – 40.

[63] McMurray RG, Hicks LL, Thompson DL. The effects of passive inhalation of cigarette smoke on exercise performance. *Eur. J. Appl. Physiol.* 1985; 54: 196 – 200.

[64] Pimm PE, Silverman F, Shepard RJ. Physiolgical effects of acute passive exposure to cigarette smoke. *Arch. Environ. Healt.* 1978; 33: 201 – 13.

[65] Lough J. Cardiomyopathy produced by cigarette smoke. Ultrastructural observations in guinea pigs. *Arch. Pathol. Lab. Med.* 1978: 102: 377 – 80.

[66] *Smoking and Health. Report of the Surgeon General.* US Department of Health, Education, and Welfare. 1979.

[67] Leone A. The heart:a target organ for cigarette smoking. *J. Smoking-Related Dis.* 1992; 3: 197 – 201.

[68] Leone A, Lopez M, Picerno G. Il ruolo del fumo nel determinismo della cardiopatia coronarica. *Min. Cardiang.* 1984; 32: 435 – 9.

Chapter 3

Gross and Microscopic Anatomy of Structures Involved

Abstract

Gross, microscopic and ultrastructural characteristics of those structures of heart and vessel affected by passive smoking are analyzed.

Myocardium is composed primarily of a collection of branching and specialized striated muscle cells (cardiac myocytes), and a series of other structures related to myocytes: sarcolemma, sarcoplastic reticulum, contractile proteins, mitochondria and nucleus. A fibrous skeleton supports cardiac framework.

Coronary arteries, named left main coronary artery with its branches – left anterior descending artery and circumflex artery – and right coronary artery, supply the heart of blood according, physiologically, to its metabolic necessities.

Endothelium is a metabolically active lining structure of the vessels and heart (endocardium) that is affected early functionally by smoking exposure. Its functional alterations, simply defined as endothelial dysfunction, usually precede the appearance of anatomical changes in this structure.

There is evidence that the negative effects of passive smoking particularly alter some cardiovascular sites which have a major affinity with smoking toxics as well as more active metabolic functions.

Keywords: Anatomy, Myocardium, Coronary arteries, Vascular Endothelium, Heart examination.

Since both a hypoxic mechanism and direct damage due to passive smoking compounds cause those structural alterations of cardiovascular system that usually have been well identified, the obvious consequence is that there is a basic involvement of their anatomy that will be evident after prolonged chronic exposure, whereas prevailingly functional disorders follow acute exposure. Among affected structures, particularly myocardium, namely cardiac muscle cells, coronary arteries, intramyocardial vessels, and vascular endothelium are the target organ of passive smoke. Indeed, these structures are those which particularly feel hypoxia as well as changes in blood flow and blood components [1–3] capable to induce cellular alterations and atherosclerotic lesion progression [4–7].

In this chapter, gross and microscopic characteristics of contractile myocardial muscle cells, extramural coronary arteries and intramyocardial vessels as well as normal endothelium are reviewed in an attempt to a better understand those changes that they meet as a consequence of environmental tobacco smoke exposure.

CONTRACTILE MYOCARDIUM

Myocardium is the supporting structure of the heart together with fibrous cardiac skeleton. Heart function is a result of the myocardial integrity since the other cardiac structures such as cardiac valves, endocardium, which is the endothelial lining of the heart, and pericardium are structures deputed to control blood stream direction and viscosity as well as diastolic cardiac expansion.

Myocardial contractility determines the amount of arterial blood flow that is distributed peripherically. It comes out the blood of the previous cardiac filling as a consequence of intracardiac pressure levels existing through atrial and ventricular cavities of the heart during the different phases of cardiac cycle.

Schematically, cardiac contractility needs oxygen supplied by coronary arteries. Moreover, the amount of oxygen varies according to the working demand of heart that continuously changes in relation to the metabolic requests of different tissues and organs of the body. Therefore, there is evidence that a decrease in oxygen availability causes an impairment of cardiac function with, in the long run, structural alterations of those constituents of cardiac muscle cells that particularly suffer because of the reduced amount in oxygen.

Several factors (Table 3.1.) modulate cardiac contractility [8], but oxygen availability is believed to be one of the most important.

Table 3.1. Main factors which modulate cardiac contractility

Oxygen availability
Beta adrenergic stimulation
Calcium ions and Tubular calcium channels
Sodium /Calcium changes
Molecular status of contractile proteins (troponin C, titin, actin, myosin)

The knowledge of the gross, microscopic, and ultrastructural characteristics of myocardium are the basis to interpret correctly the type of alterations caused by passive smoking on the heart.

Grossly, myocardium (Figure 3.1.) consists of muscular fibers which are attached to a fibrous ring. Myocardium is closely covered by the visceral layer of the serous pericardium, named epicardium, whereas its cavities are lined by the endocardium. Between these two structures, there is the muscular wall of the heart that is, in the strict sense of the word, the myocardium.

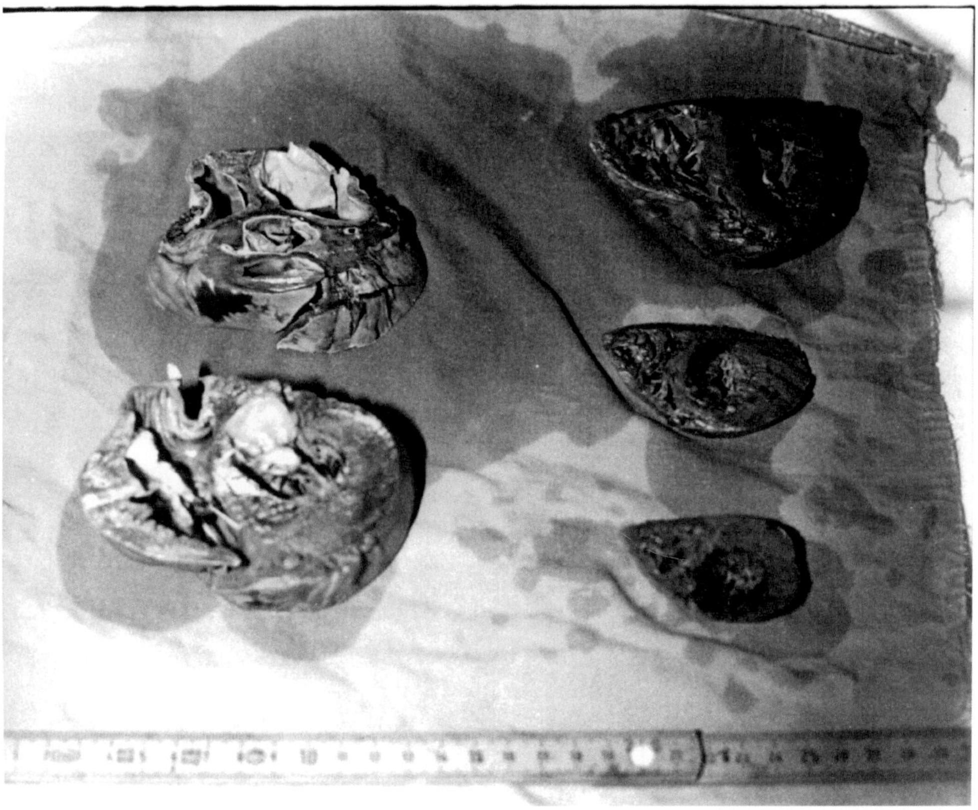

Figure 3.1. Gross examination of the heart according to Roussy and Ameuille technique [29]. Parallel slices of about 1 cm in thickness are conducted from the base to the apex of the heart.

It consists of bands of fibers which have an intricately complex interlacement, crossing each other according to an order due to their function. They are of a deep red color and marked with transverse striae. There are muscular fibers for atrial wall and muscular fibers for the ventricles which are much thicker than those of the atria (left ventricular wall thickness is about from 13 to 16 millimeter tick versus 4 – 6 millimeters of left atrium thickness) and also quite independent of other ones with regard to their function and anatomical significance. Such a difference is to be kept carefully in mind since it clearly explains the reasons of the different localization of myocardial alterations from hypoxia due to environmental tobacco smoke as well as other hypoxic factors. Thus, the work of those structures anatomically thicker demands a major oxygen supply which could still be insufficient because of the hypoxic mechanisms. Therefore, cardiac alterations affect particularly the ventricles being the atrial wall partly spared for both less wall thickness and anatomical and functional property to be independent from the function of the ventricles.

These gross characteristics are consistent with microscopic and ultrastructural patterns of contractile myocardium, although several different types of cells may be recognized into the cardiac muscle particuarly related to the impulse formation and its conduction [9]. These last cells are located primarily along the conduction system and usually are not affected by passive smoking. That is true as far as ventricular arrhythmias in patients with a previous myocardial infarction after exposure to passive smoking [10] are a consequence of contractile myocardium alterations rather than alterations of specific conduction system of the heart.

Therefore, histological and ultrastructural characteristics of contractile myocardium, usually related to possible damage due to environmental tobacco smoke exposure, will be briefly described.

Histologically (Figures 3.2. and 3.3.), contractile myocardium is composed of a network of branching striated muscle cells with centrally located nuclei. A plasma membrane named sarcolemma surrounds each cell which contains a series of long parallel myofibrils with a regular direction, namely the contractile substance of the heart muscle, and such a structure gives a striated appearance to the muscle fibers. The fibers are separated from one another by intracellular spaces, which are of different width and contain small amount of collagen, occasional fibroblasts and numerous capillaries, which form a consistent end-part of the intramural circulation of the myocardium and flow together into the intramural venular framework that will empty on outside metabolized nutritional substances previously used for the energetic pathways of myocardial cells.

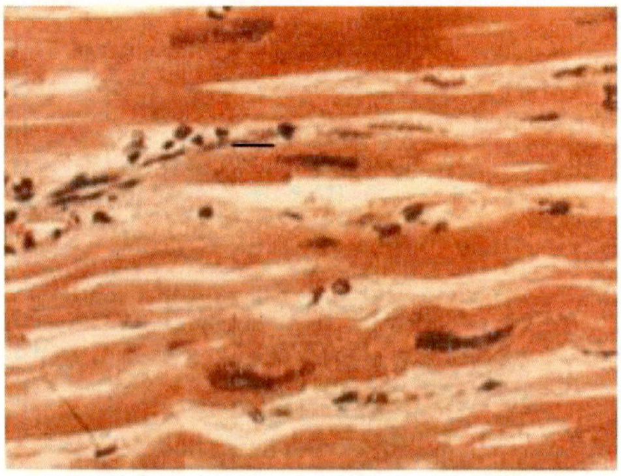

Figure 3.2. Histologic pattern of Myocardium.

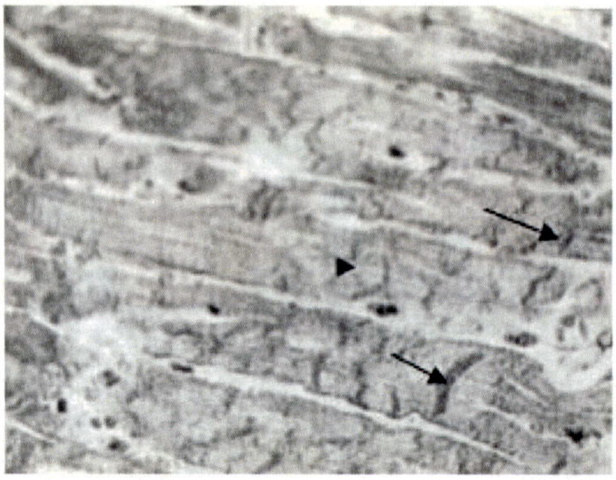

Figure 3.3. Histologic pattern of myocardium External zone of a human infarct with numerous contraction bands (arrows).

The knowledge of these structures must be kept in mind since carbon monoxide can directly affect these sites, causing some of those lesions that are integral part of toxic cardiomyopathy [11–13]. Minute pinocytotic vesicles are present along the cytoplasmic surface of the muscle cells as well as mitochondria, ribosomes and RNA –dependent components that may be all involved negatively in prolonged chronic exposure to passive smoking although with either a different degree of damage or appearance.

Ultrastructurally (Figures 3.4, 3.5, and 3.6.), observations on the characteristics of myocardium arise particularly from animal models. Moreover, the ultrastructural lesions related to smoking exposure have been studied experimentally in animals [14–16].

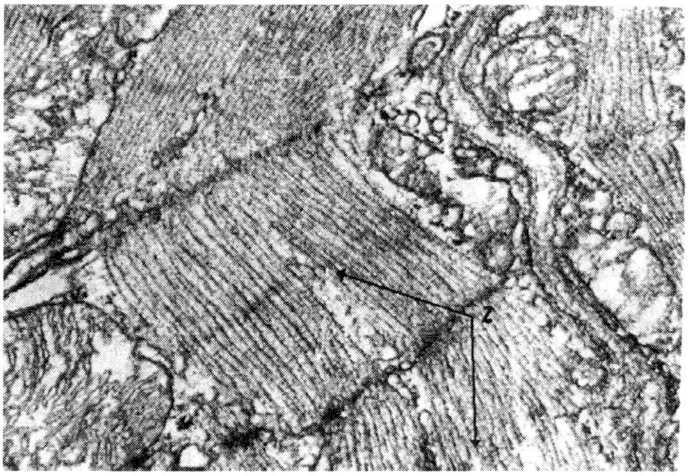

Figure 3.4. Ultrastructural myocardium showing cardiocytes with myofilaments and Z bands. Outside the cardiocytes, there is a deeply altered structure of cardiac muscle.

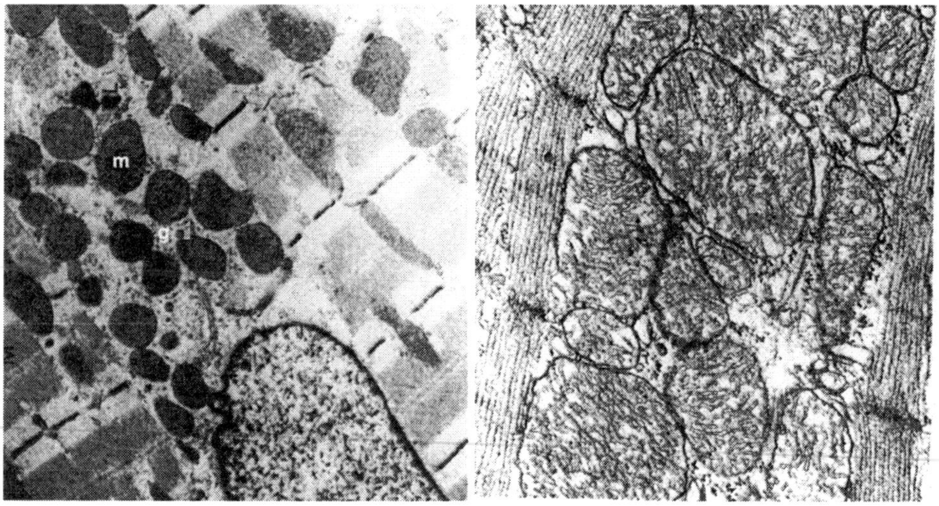

Figures 3.5. and 3.6. Normal cardiocytes in longitudinal section showing regular myofilaments, mitochondria (m), lysosomes, and a few glicogen granules (g).

Contractile myocardial cell is about 100 μm long and 15 μm wide. At its end, each cell takes on contact with adjacent myocardial cells. An intercalated disk with gap junctions is placed at the cell ends and it allows a close anatomical and functional contact among the different myocytes. An extracellular space contains a complex network of myocardial cells which are closely related to a capillary network. The basic units of contraction are the sarcomeres that are aligned at Z line in adjacent myofibrils. They give the characteristically striated appearance to the heart muscle. Each myocardial cell is surronded by a membrane, named sarcolemma, particularly rich in lipids and proteins. Each myocardial cell also has T-tubules, which are invaginations from the cell surface going regularly down to each Z-line in each myofibril, and a sarcoplasmic reticulum. All these structures are deputed to provide ion and electrical flow as well as the necessary energy to permit sarcomere contraction. Energy for contraction comes from mitochondria, that are about one and third in volume of myofibrils, through metabolic pathways involving adenosine triphosphate (ATP). These structures are closely dependent on each other, clearly explain the reason for altered contraction due to chronically prolonged smoking exposure, although the chemical compounds of smoke act particularly only on some of them. Moreover, each sarcomere contains two interdigitating filaments: the tick filament is made of the protein myosin, and the thin filament is made of actin. These molecules are the specific contractile material. Contraction is the result of sliding of the thin actin filaments relative to the tick myosin filaments without any shortening of themselves, the length of which remains constant [17–22], with the breakdown of ATP. Another protein, the Troponin, strictly attached to actin molecules, initiates the contraction after its binding with calcium.

These concise data about the close relationship among all different components of myocardial cells provide material for better understanding the type and complex way of myocardial damage due to smoke exposure.

Coronary Arteries and Intramural Circulation

A description of the main characteristics of extramural and intramural circulation of the coronary arteries set together to explain possible different mechanisms which can cause cardiovascular damage due to passive smoking exposure. Also in this case, the phenomenon is related to hypoxia linked with anatomical and/or functional changes affecting vessel structures usually with a reduction in lumen diameter because of presence of isolated or multiple stenoses of different size and degree.

Extramural Coronary Arteries

The coronary arteries arise within the sinuses of Valsalva behind the aortic valve leaflets. Most of the coronary artery filling occurs during cardiac diastole. There are two main coronary arteries: the left main coronary arteries which, after a short distance, branches into two vessels, respectively the anterior descending artery and the circumflex artery, and the right coronary artery. Functionally, the coronary arteries are as end arteries, although anatomically numerous intercoronary and intracoronary anastomoses exist up to 40 μm in diameter in most normal hearts.

The knowledge of what myocardial area is supplied by coronary arteries needs to explain both the localization and course of myocardium alterations as well as the relationship between vascular lesions and degree of cardiac lesions.

A detailed analysis of the anatomy of the coronary tree is beyond the purpose of this book. On the contrary, it is basic to know coronary flow distribution to heart muscle.

The anterior descending artery of the left coronary artery particularly supplies the anterior wall of the left ventricle, the bordering third of the anterior surface of the right ventricle, the anterior two-thirds of the interventricular septum and most of the heart apex.

The right coronary artery supplies the reminder wall of right ventricle anteriorly and posteriorly, the posterior third of both the left ventricular wall and interventricular septum.

Finally, the circumflex artery, after its origin from the left coronary artery, supplies a small portion of the lateral myocardium of the left ventricle together with a small portion of left ventricle anteriorly and posteriorly.

The course and branching of coronary arteries may be shown in a postmortem coronary angiography (Figure 3.7.) [23–24].

Intramural Circulation

Intramyocardial circulation is formed by: 1. Intramyocardial coronary arteries; 2. Coronary arterioles; 3. Intercoronary and intracoronary anastomoses; 4. Capillary bed.

It's either the anatomical integrity of extramural coronary arteries or myocardial mass since these vessels are respectively stressed and released during systole and diastole of cardiac cycle. In cases of poor availability in oxygen, intramyocardial vessels suffer chronically and show in time hyperplastic and degenerative changes with evident impairment of their metabolic function. The basic function of intramural circulation is also to provide anastomoses among adjacent branches. These anastomoses can undergo a gradual enlargement or also become functionally of significant caliber if their wall does not show alterations. Finally, intramural vessels branch into a capillary bed and may be connected directly with cardiac chambers as arterioluminal vessels [25–27]

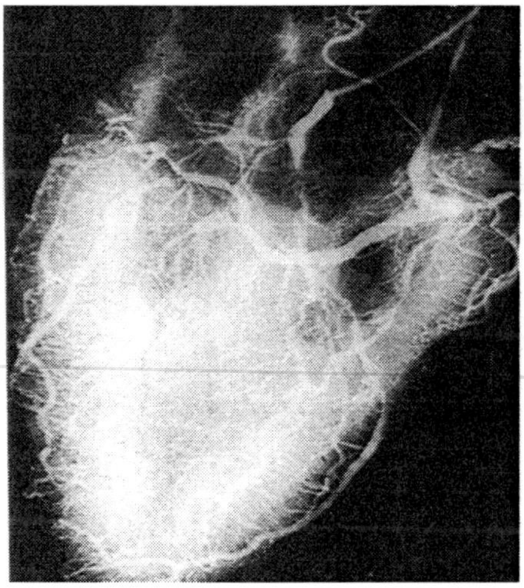

Figure 3.7: Postmortem coronary angiography showing the distribution of the coronary tree. A radiopaque mass fills the four major coronary arteries as well as its branches. A rich intramural framework with small vessel anastomoses and capillary bed may be also observed.

Atrial Circulation

The atria are supplied by small branches arising from the coronary trunks of the corresponding side.

Pathological narrowings or occlusion of the coronary arteries can cause severe damage to ventricular muscle, but much less to atrial muscle. Therefore, those myocardial lesions due to passive smoking prefer a ventricular localization rather than an atrial site.

Gross and Microscopic Study of the Heart

Gross and microscopic study of the heart has been conducted by using the technique proposed by Virchow [28]. It permits an useful examination of the gross characteristics of cardiac muscle, but poor results are recorded for the coronary arteries. On the contrary, a more complete study of the postmortem characteristics of the heart and coronary tree may be obtained by the technique of the serial slices of the heart described by Roussy and Ameuille [29]. This method must be preceded by an injection of radiopaque material into the coronary tree by either using different techniques or radiopaque mass with different chemical composition [23, 30].

Technically, the heart [30] is removed by severing the pulmonary artery and aorta about 5 cm from the free margin of the semilunar valves. After observing the external aspect of the heart to identify possible areas of myocardial damage, without opening the coronary vessels, a plug is placed through the aorta into the aortic orifice and then the coronary arteries are injected at a pressure of 130 mmHg using a barium-iodine-gelatin radiopaque mass by a cannula tied into the aorta. When a good degree of contrast is noted in X-rays, the heart is fixed in 10 percent formalin- water solution and then cut into 5 to 6 transverse slices of approximately 1 cm in thickness from the apex to the base. These slices are parallel to each other and atrio-ventricular sulcus. The thickness of the left ventricular wall is conventionally measured at the level of the third slice. If lesions of the cardiac muscle are seen, they are quantified in percent by a comparison to the total myocardium from the photographs by means of a polar planimeter.

Every major coronary artery and its branches are cut transversely along their length at an interval of approximately 5 mm. If alterations are seen, their length and degree is recorded.

Microscopic examination of the myocardium and coronary arteries is carried out by using standard staining, particularly hematoxylin-eosin. For the myocardium pieces to be studied, possible damaged areas are observed grossly, around its borders and at different levels of normal myocardium. For the coronary arteries, each removed segment is studied microscopically with about more than 100 segments examined per heart [31]. At light microscopy, these structures are analyzed and possible narrowings of the coronary arteries measured with an ocular micrometer and then recorded.

This method of study provides data on almost the total myocardium as well as coronary tree.

To use this method, some equipments as well as chemical reagents to prepare the radiopaque mass need.

Firstly, an equipment for standard x-rays should complete the autopsy room.

Among chemicals, barium sulfate, bacto-gelatins, iodine preparation for angiographic injection, and cannulae of different size are the material that must be used to prepare radiopaque mass [30].

VASCULAR ENDOTHELIUM

The vascular endothelium has been long interpreted as a simply physical separation between blood and tissue [32] , a lining of the arterial intima to protect passively this structure from the mechanical injuries coming through the blood.

Over the last twenty years, experimental and clinical results experienced that endothelium is not only a lining structure of vessels and heart (endocardium), but particularly a widely distributed organ among and within tissues [33–34] deeply involved to regulate vascular physiology and its pathophysiologic changes. These functions are strictly related to its position at the interface between blood and tissue. Moreover, the progression of the knowledge on endothelial function has demonstrated that, similarly to the heart [35]), the endothelium can also be considered a target organ of the exposure to passive smoking [36–41], that is capable to induce earlier endothelial dysfunction and, then later, after several years, structural alterations.

There is growing evidence that endothelium, among the different structures of the body, is capable to better harmonize its anatomical shape with function. Therefore, early endothelial dysfunction may induce alterations that are the "door" of vascular changes that are responsible, of atherosclerotic and thrombotic pathology [42–44]. Thus, analyzing functional endothelial response could be kept in mind before searching for anatomical alterations. In the presence of a physiologic response of endothelium, anatomical changes in this structure are usually lacking.

Anatomically, endothelium is composed of a single layer of poligonal, elongated cells joined edge to edge forming junctional complexes with adjacent cells. Inside the cells there is a large number of pinocytotic vesicles that are consistent with functional patterns. This particular structure of endothelium forms an unique membrane of cells which represent the storage organelle for von Willebrand factor, a complex protein with procoagulant activity, the deficiency of which causes classic hemophilia [45], and interferes with all those factors which are involved to build the Virchow's triad in thrombosis [46] (Figure 3.8.). Its main factor is represented, as Virchow precisely described, by an injury capable to alter structurally the endothelium and by doing so, trigger a mechanism for a possible development of thrombosis. Nowdays, there is evidence that functional alterations of the endothelium (endothelial dysfunction) can have the same effect.

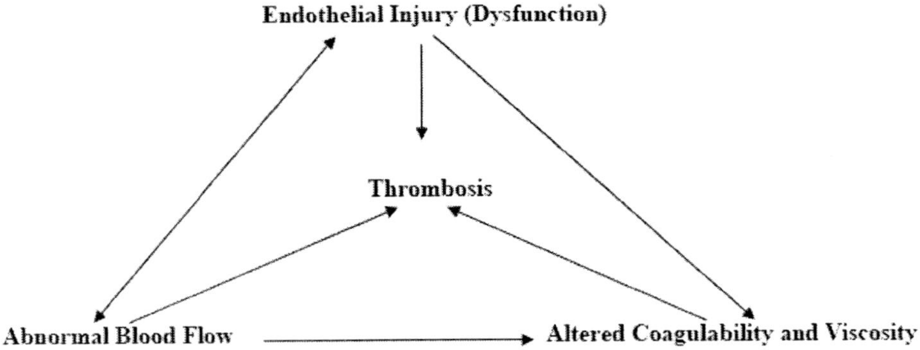

Figure 3.8 Virchow's triad in thrombosis. Endothelial integrity is the basic factor to avoid a triggering mechanism for thrombus formation. Injured endothelial cells can trigger an abnormal blood viscosity and consequent hypercoagulability which can activate the thrombus-formation via.

Vascular endothelium is recognized to be a tissue with multifunctional properties the main of which are listed in Table 3.2.

Table 3.2. Endothelial cells functional and metabolic properties

Property	Function
1. Semipermeable barrier	Modulates the transfer of molecules into the arterial wa
2. Elaboration of antithrombotic molecules	Regulates thrombosis, thrombolysis, and platelet adherence
3. Tissue factors	Modulates vascular tone and blood flow
4. Metabolic effects on hormone synthesis	
5. Immunologic and inflammatory reaction	Leukocyte interactions with vessels
6. Lipid metabolism interference	Modifies lipoproteins in arterial wall
7. Smooth muscle cells	Regulates growing, physiologic tone, and shape

Particularly, the coagulation thrombosis cascade, vascular tone, inflammatory and immunologic reactions are modulated by endothelial cell integrity [32, 47–48]. Thus, as firstly reported by Furchgott and Zawadzki [49], there is certain evidence of a primary autocrine/paracrine regulatory role of endothelial cells in secreting substances that control both vascular tone and structure. Indeed, vascular tone is the function primarily altered by endothelial dysfunction following passive smoking exposure, being an anatomical structure of endothelial cells, also negatively affected later.

Endothelium produces [50] several relaxing factors including nitric oxide and prostacyclin as well as endothelium-derived contracting factors – cyclooxygenase-dependent contracting factors and endothelin 1 – which, physiologically, act to regulate functional integrity of endothelial cells and particularly, cardiovascular responses.

Endothelium-derived nitric oxide is one of the most investigated substances secreted by endothelium [51]. It is a potent vasodilator, inhibits platelet aggregation, vascular smooth muscle cell migration and proliferation, and monocyte adhesion. By this way, arterial wall maintains its physiological properties and is protected against the development of atherosclerosis [49–51]. It is worth to observe that impaired nitric oxide availability potentiates all those major risk factors which can be associated with atherosclerosis [52–55] appearance or progression.

If endothelium is intact, its stimulation causes vascular dilatation since there are prevailing effects of the relaxing substances. On the contrary, an enhanced vasoconstrictor activity is the result of impaired nitric oxide availability with a loss of endothelial-dependent vasodilation that characterizes endothelial dysfunction, an early but initially reversible sign in healthy individuals due, among other things, to environmental tobacco smoke. Endothelial dysfunction may be followed by a series of active processes such as inflammation, proliferation or apoptosis. Thus, damage of the endothelium leads to an endothelial activation, the final result of which is appearance and/or progression of an atherosclerotic plaque that can be considered as an expression of an anatomical damage.

In conclusion, integrity of the endothelium keeps vascular homeostasis and prevents cardiovascular damage. On the contrary, endothelial dysfunction must be carefully avoided since it is the door of a large series of alterations that are particularly harmful for cardiovascular system. Indeed, passive smoking, as aforesaid, is an early and impending factor of endothelial dysfunction.

Finally, as previously underlined, anatomical alterations of the endothelial cells follow far functional disorders of these structures. Therefore, the observation of endothelial cells anatomically intact is not necessarily evidence of endothelium integrity. Such a fact must be kept in mind when people exposed to passive smoking are investigated.

Are There Characteristics that Explain the Alterations in Some Structures ?

From the appearances, the localization of the lesions affecting some anatomical structures rather than others of cardiovascular system could seem to occur by chance. On the contrary, there are evident reasons that explain the choice of specific anatomical targets for the chemical components of passive smoking. These reasons correlate with the type of physiopathologic mechanism of damage. Indeed, three mechanisms of cardiovascular damage due to passive smoking may occur: a hypoxic mechanism, direct damage of chemical toxics on some structures rather than others, and a combined action of both these mechanisms.

There is evidence that the physiological properties of anatomical structures of cardiovascular system can have more negative influences when a damaging stimulus tends to change their function.

Therefore, some questions, that need explanation and can be explained, arise: which structures feel a major rate with the hypoxic mechanism? Which with the direct damage? Which with the combined mechanisms? Why? How are they affected? The answers to these questions are possibly analyzing the link between the biological characteristics of the anatomical constituents and chemical compounds of passive smoking.

Hypoxia is a strong cause of cell injury consisting, specifically, of a reduced intracellular oxygen availability of different degree, which depends on the characteristic of the responsible factor. Oxygen is the most important substance that allows regularly intracellular respiratory changes since it is the terminal receptor of all metabolic substances produced by intracellular nutrition. The end result of cellular metabolism is forming water and carbon dioxide to the production of which oxygen actively contributes. Carbon dioxide is then removed by extracellular venous return.

Respiratory metabolism in living cells serves particularly two functions: to provide energy for cellular vital processes and transform dietary material into cellular constituents [56].

Those intracellular structures deputed to develop these function are RNA-related constituents, particularly mitochondria, that receive from the cytoplasm oxidizable substrates that will be addressed to intracellular metabolic chains. From that, there is evidence from intracellular localization of myocardial damage due to passive smoking, as well as involvement of those structures as ventricular muscle cells, that have major metabolic requests to develop their function.

Moreover, depending from the severity of hypoxia, the cells may adapt with chronic suffering, undergo acute injury, or die. The last occurence needs other factors, particularly ischemia that causes reduction or loss of blood supply as a consequence of progression of atherosclerotic lesions or plaque rupture, particularly if there is endothelial dysfunction.

To what concerns carboxyhemoglobin, similar observations can be carried out, considering the direct damage that carbon monoxide may produce on myocardial cells.

Loss of the oxygen-carrying capacity of the blood due to binding between carbon monoxide and hemoglobin that blocks oxygen carriage is not only due to the affinity of about 240 times major of hemoglobin for the gas but also to its environmental levels.

Moreover, the type of lesions that carbon monoxide is capable of to cause directly in different organs and tissues has major affinity for some anatomical sites, particularly heart and vessels [57], and in the context of these structures cardiac muscle cells, interstitium, and vascular endothelium [58-59].

It is noteworthy that carbon monoxide, besides to bind hemoglobin and thus, induce hypoxia, is also capable of binding to muscle myoglobin [35] and interferes negatively with oxygen availability to intracellular mitochondria. It can also affect cytochrome oxidase system into cellular cytoplasm impairing all intracellular oxidative reactions. If binding with myoglobin or negative interference with oxidative enzymes is strong in amount, the function and anatomical structures of the cardiac muscle cells can be heavily altered in those components with major affinity towards this toxic gas.

In conclusion, there exist both anatomical and functional characteristics that explain the localization of cardiovascular damage due to passive smoking in those structures that particularly have a chemical affinity with smoking toxics.

The anatomical characteristics of those structures particularly affected by environmental tobacco exposure are noteworthy since that allows a clarification of either the mechanisms of the lesions or their appearance in time. As already described chemical structure of smoking toxics, which may have open chemical chains, determines the possibility of chemical reactions between these compounds and compounds of those cellular structures where metabolic changes occur continuously to ensure, physiologically, cell living. It needs chemical reactions that can be disturbed by all those chemicals which may interfere at different metabolic steps.

REFERENCES

[1] Leone A. Cardiovascular damage from smoking: a fact or belief? *Int J Cardiol* 1993; 38: 113 – 7.

[2] Hammond EC, Garfinkel L. Coronary heart disease, stroke and aortic aneurysm. *Arch Environ Health* 1969; 19: 167 – 82.

[3] Auerbach O, Carter HW, Garfinkel M, Hammond EC. Cigarette smoking and coronary heart disease, a macroscopic and microscopic study. *Chest* 1976; 70: 697 – 705.

[4] Leone A, Lopez M. Oral contraception, ovarian disorders and tobacco in myocardial infarction of woman. *Pathologica* 1986; 78: 237 – 42.

[5] Strong JP, Richards ML. Cigarette smoking and atherosclerosis in autopsied men. *Atherosclerosis* 1976; 23: 451 – 76.

[6] Auerbach O, Hammond EC, Garfinkel L. Smoking in ralation to atherosclerosis of the coronary arteries. *New Engl J Med* 1965; 273: 775 – 9.

[7] Glantz SA, Parmley WW. Passive smoking and heart disease. *JAMA* 1995; 273: 1047 – 53.

[8] Opie LH. Mechanisms of cardiac contraction and relaxation. In : *Braunwald's Heart Disease. A Textbook of Cardiovascular Medicine*; Zipes DP, Libby P, Bonow RO, Braunwald E eds., Elsevier-Saunders , Philadelphia, Pennsylvania, USA; 2005: 457 – 89.

[9] James TN. The connecting pathways between the sinus node and the A-V node and between the right and left atrium in the human heart. *Am Heart J* 1963; 66: 498 – 508.

[10] Leone A, Bertanelli F, Mori L, Fabiano P, Bertoncini G. Ventricular arrhythmias by passive smoke in patients with pre-existing myocardial infarction. *J Am Coll Cardiol* 1992; 3: 256 A.

[11] Marius-Nunez AL. Myocardial infarction with normal coronary arteries after acute exposure to carbon monoxide. *Chest* 1990; 97: 491 – 4.

[12] Roberts JR, Bain M, Klachko MN, Seigel EG, Wason S. Successful heart transplantation from a victim of carbon monoxide poisoning. *Ann Emerg Med* 1995; 26: 652 – 5.

[13] Astrup P. The arterial wall in atherogenesis. In *Atherogenesis*, Cavallero C ed; Piccin Medical Book, Padua, Italy 1965; 77- 92.

[14] Lough J. Cardiomyopathy produced by cigarette smoke. Ultrastructural observations in guinea pigs. Arch Pathol Lab Med 1978; 102: 377 – 80.

[15] Kjeldsen K, Thomsen HK, Astrup P. Effects of carbon monoxide on myocardium. Ultrastructural changes in rabbits after moderate, chronic exposure. *Circ Res* 1974; 34: 339 – 48.

[16] DeBias DA, Banerjee CM, Birkhead NC, Harrer WV, Kazal LA. Carbon monoxide inhalation effects following myocardial infarction in monkeys. *Arch Environ Health* 1973; 27: 161 – 7.

[17] Huxley HE. The double array of filaments in cross-striated muscle. *J Biophys Biochem Cytol* 1957; 3: 631 – 48.
[18] Huxley AF. Muscle structure and theories of contraction. *Progr Biophys* 1957; 7: 255 – 318.
[19] Huxley AF, Niedergerke R. Structural changes in muscle during contraction. Interference microscopy of living muscle fibers. *Nature* 1954; 173: 971 – 3.
[20] Huxley AF, Taylor RE. Local activation of striated muscle fibers. *J Physiol* 1958; 144: 426 – 41.
[21] Huxley HE. The contractile structure of cardiac and skeletal muscle. *Circulation* 1961; 24: 328 – 35.
[22] Huxley HE, Hanson J. Changes in the cross-striations of muscle during contraction and stretch and their structural interpretation. *Nature* 1954; 173; 973 – 6.
[23] Schlesinger MJ. An injection plus dissection study of coronary artery occlusions and anastomoses. *Am Heart J* 1938; 15: 528 – 68.
[24] Salans AH, Tweed P. A preliminary study of the coronary circulation post-mortem. *Am Heart J* 1947; 33: 477 – 89.
[25] Wearn JT. The extent of the capillary bed of the heart. *J Exp Med* 1928; 47: 273 – 91.
[26] Wearn JT. The role of the thebesian vessels in the circulation of the heart. *J Exp Med* 1928; 47: 293 – 316.
[27] Wearn JT, Mettier SR, Klump TG, Zschiesche LJ. The nature of the vascular communications between the coronary arteries and the chambers of the heart. *Am Heart J* 1933; 9: 143 – 64.
[28] Virchow R. *Postmortem examination with especial references to medico-legal practice* Bakiston Sons, Philadelphia, Pennsylvania, USA, 1896: 143 – 7.
[29] Roussy G, Ameuille P. *Technique des autopsies et des recherches anatomo-pathologiques à l'Amphitheatre.* O Doin et Fills, Paris 1910.
[30] Leone A. L'angiografia coronarica postmortem nello studio anatomo-patologico del cuore. *Giorn It Card* 1972; 2: 688 – 92.
[31] Baroldi G, Radice F, Schmid G, Leone A. Morphology of acute myocardial infarction in relation to coronary thrombosis. *Am Heart J* 1974; 87: 65 – 75.
[32] Fishman AP. Endothelium: a distributed organ of diverse capabilities. *Ann NY Acad Sci* 1982; 401: 1 – 8.
[33] Cines DB, Pollak ES, Buck CA, Loscalzo J, Zimmerman GA, McEver RP, Pober JS, Wick TM, Konkle BA, Schwartz BS, Barnathan ES, McCrae KR, Hug BA, Schmidt AM, Stern DM. Endothelial cells in physiology and in the pathophysiology of vascular disorders. *Blood* 1998; 91: 3527 – 61.
[34] Stevens T, Rosemberg R, Aird W, Quertenous T, Johnson FL, Garcia JG, Hebbel RP, Tuder RM, Garfinkel S. NHLBI workshop report : endothelial cell phenotypes in heart, lung, and blood diseases. *Am J Physiol Cell Physiol* 2001; 281: C1422 – 33.
[35] Leone A. The heart: a target organ for cigarette smoking. *J Smoking-Related Dis* 1992; 3: 197 – 201.
[36] Celermajer DS, Adams MR, Clarkson P, Robinson J, McRedie R, Donald A, Deanfield JE. Passive smoking and impaired endothelium-dependent arterial dilatation in healthy young adults. *N Engl J Med* 1996; 334: 150 – 4.

[37] Sumida H, Watanabe H, Kugiyama K, Ohgushi M, Matsumura T, Yasue H. Does passive smoking impair endothelium-dependent coronary artery dilation in women? *J Am Coll Cardiol* 1998; 31: 811 – 5.

[38] Davis J, Shelton L, Watanabe I, Arnold J. Passive smoking affects endothelium and platelets. *Arch Intern Med* 1989; 149: 386 – 9.

[39] Raitakari OT, Adams MR, McRedie RJ, Griffiths KA, Celermajer DS. Passive-smoke related arterial endothelial dysfunction is potentially reversible in healthy young adults. *Ann Intern Med* 1999; 130: 578 – 81.

[40] Celermajer DS, Sorensen KE, Georgakopoulos D. Cigarette smoking is associated with dose-related and potentially reversible impairment of endothelium-dependent dilation in healthy young adults. *Circulation* 1993; 88: 2149 – 55.

[41] Deedwania PC. Endothelium: a new target for cardiovascular therapeutics. *J Am Coll Cardiol* 2000; 35: 67 – 70.

[42] Desideri GB, Ferri C. Endothelial activation. Sliding door to atherosclerosis. *Curr Pharm Design* 2005; 11: 2163 – 75.

[43] Taddei S, Ghiadoni L, Virdis A, Versari D, Salvetti A. Mechanisms of endothelial dysfunction: clinical significance and preventive non-pharmacological therapeutic strategies. *Curr Pharm Design* 2003; 9: 2385 – 402.

[44] Libby P. Inflammation in atherosclerosis. Nature 2002; 420: 868 – 74.

[45] Nemerson Y, Williams WJ. Biochemistry of plasma coagulation factors. In *Hematology,* William WJ, Beutler E, Erslev AJ, Lichtman MA eds., McGraw-Hill Publishing Company, 4th ed, New York et al, USA, 1990: 1267 – 84.

[46] Virchow RL. Beitr Z exp *Pathol* 1846; 2: 227 – 380.

[47] Frenette PS, Wagner DD. Adhesion molecules. *N Engl J Med* 1996; 334: 1526 – 9.

[48] Frenette PS, Wagner DD. Adhesion molecules-blood vessels and blood cells. *N Engl J Med* 1996; 335: 43 – 5.

[49] Furchgott RF, Zawadzki JV. The obligatory role of endothelial cells in the relaxation of arterial smooth muscle by acetylcholine. *Nature* 1980; 288: 373 – 6.

[50] Luscher TF, Vanhouette PM. *The endothelium: modulator of cardiovascular function.* 1990, Boca Raton: CRC Press.

[51] Palmer RM, Ferrige AG, Moncada S. Nitric oxide release accounts for the biological activity of endothelium-derived relaxing factor. *Nature* 1987; 327: 524 – 6.

[52] Stroes ES, Koomans HA, de Bruin TW, Rabelink TJ. Vascular function in the forearm of hypercholesterolaemic patients off and on lipid-lowering medication. *Lancet* 1995; 346: 467 – 71.

[53] Panza JA, Garcia CE, Kilcoyne CM, Quyyumi AA, Cannon RO. Impaired endothelium-dependent vasodilation in patients with essential hypertension. Evidence that nitric-oxide abnormality is not localized to a single signal transduction pathway. *Circulation* 1995; 91: 1732 – 8.

[54] Johnstone MT, Creager SJ, Scales KM, Cusco JA, Lee BK, Creager MA. Impaired endothelium-dependent vasodilation in patients with insulin-dependent diabetes mellitus. *Circulation* 1993; 88: 2510 – 6.

[55] Ting HH, Timimi FK, Boles KS, Creager SJ, Ganz P, Creager MA. Vitamin C improves endothelium-dependent vasodilation in patients with non-insulin-dependent diabetes mellitus. *J Clin Invest* 1996; 97: 22 – 8.

[56] White A, Handler P, Smith EL. Biological Oxidations II. In *Principles of Biochemistry*, White A, Handler P, Smith EL eds., 4th ed, McGraw-Hill Book Company , New York, Sidney, Toronto, London; 1968; 321 – 54.

[57] Anderson EW, Andelman RJ, Strauch JM, Fortuin NJ, Knelson JH. Effect of low-level carbon monoxide exposure on onset and duration of angina pectoris. *Ann Intern Med* 1973; 79: 46 – 50.

[58] Coburn RF. Mechanisms of carbon monoxide toxicity. *Preventive Medicine* 1979; 8: 310 – 22.

[59] Valkonen M, Kuusi T. Passive smoking induces atherogenic changes in low-density lipoprotein. *Circulation* 1998: 97: 2012 – 6.

Chapter 4

STRUCTURAL DISORDERS OF CARDIOVASCULAR SYSTEM

ABSTRACT

Structural changes that affect cardiovascular system as a consequence of passive smoking exposure do not differ from those attributable to the same disease caused by other factors, although some differences may be met in the development and manifestations of the lesion when both active or passive smoking are the responsible factors.

Atherosclerosis development and progression with fibrous plaque formation, followed sometimes by complications such as thrombosis, plaque rupture with distal embolization and hemorrhage, are the most important alterations closely related to passive smoking. These alterations are the consequence of repeated functional events, particularly endothelial dysfunction and sympathetic stimulation, that are a common response to passive smoking exposure in each exposed individual. They can also trigger atherosclerotic process that is usually a late manifestation of passive smoking.

Coronary heart disease is an event strictly related to passive smoking. Coronary atherosclerosis affects mainly the coronary arteries of both subjects suffering from stable angina and acute myocardial infarction. Moreover, in myocardial infarction, focal intramyocardial areas of hemorrhage may be seen with a major incidence when a myocardial infarction is compared with the same alteration not caused by passive smoking exposure. Severe coronary narrowings, as well as vessel calcification, usually characterize a myocardial infarction from passive smoking. Therefore, finding focal hemorrhagic zones in the context of a necrotic myocardial area, severe coronary narrowings and coronary calcification can mean that smoking exposure has influenced myocardial changes with high probability.

Other manifestations of coronary heart disease are sudden death and arrhythmias, particularly related to functional disorders induced by smoking exposure, as well as two types of cardiomyopathies: postischemic cardiomyopathy with progressive heart failure, and experimental cardiomyopathy described in different species of animals as an occurence strictly related to smoking exposure, with peculiar patterns of myocardial alterations.

Cerebrovascular disease has been well demonstrated to be a result of smoking exposure. Severe anatomical alterations associated with systemic atherosclerosis, hypertension and often, oral contraceptives in women, heavily impair the prognosis of the affected subjects.

Finally, peripheral artery disease and aortic aneurysm are manifestations for which atherosclerotic pathology and consequently, passive smoking can play a basic role. Among peripheral artery diseases, thromboangiitis obliterans is characterized either pathogenetically or pathologically by some manifestations which are typical of the disease and certainly due to a direct effect of smoking exposure or allergic mechanisms.

Keywords: Passive smoking, atherosclerosis, fibrous plaque, fibrous plaque complications, coronary heart disease, angina, myocardial infarction structural alterations, sudden death, arrhythmias, postischemic cardiomyopathy, heart enlargement, experimental cardiomyopathy, cerebrovascular disease, stroke, cerebral ischemic infarction, cerebral hemorrhagic infarction, cerebral atrophy, hypertension, peripheral artery disease, thromboangiitis obliterans, aortic aneurysm, thrombosis, emboli, rupture.

Cardiovascular pathology caused by passive smoking exposure is almost similar qualitatively to that due to active smoking, although it may differ quantitatively and with regard to its incidence [1–4].

Since a major concentration of toxic chemicals is absorbed by the smoker who smokes a cigarette while he is smoking, the longer duration in exposure to passive smoking of nonsmokers significantly reduces the difference in toxic concentration of two types of smoking which therefore act with the same mechanisms in inducing cardiovascular alterations. Moreover, the type of damage caused by smoking is similar to that caused by all other factors capable to induce the same disease, since the alterations are the result of the structural characteristics of those organs and tissues which are affected by injuries. However, differences may sometimes be documented particularly in what concerns the size and severity of the damage as well as preference in the choice of some cardiovascular structures rather than others.

Active smoking seems to cause mainly clinical and anatomical alterations related to an ischemic pathology, whereas passive smoking induces acutely functional disorders and chronically late anatomical changes related to atherosclerosis [5–8].

In Table 4.1 the pathological occurences observed with a major incidence after exposure to active smoking and passive smoking are reported.

From the analysis of Table 4.1, there is evidence of prevailing clinical signs of ischemic disease in active smokers, whereas nonsmokers passively exposed seem to suffer originally from functional disorders of cardiovascular system and later, anatomical alterations which can then cause the appearance of symptoms of a cardiovascular disease. The latter should be usually considered as a complication of an atherosclerotic lesion that may already be present without any sign of itself because of the fact that an atherosclerotic plaque is often silent up to the occurence of intercurrent events.

Table 4.1. Type of cardiovascular pathology due to both active and passive smoke

Active smoking	Passive smoking
1. Coronary artery disease (clinical and pathological signs)	1. Endothelial dysfunction
2. Stroke	2. Atherosclerosis
3. Aortic aneurysms	3. Increased heart rate
4. Cerebrovascular disease	4. Coronary heart disease
5. Peripheral vascular disease	5. Increased catecholamines
6. Changes in lipid metabolism	6. Changes in lipid metabolism
7. Hypertension	7. Cerebrovascular disease
8. Thromboangiitis obliterans	8. Hypertension
9. Sudden death	9. Arrhythmias
	10. Experimental cardiomyopathy
	11. Aortic aneurysm

To be stressed is also the change in morbidity and mortality of living beings, both smokers and nonsmokers, from cardiovascular events that seems to be well correlated statistically with smoking trend. If the trend in smoking increases, there is a major incidence of cardiovascular events. On the contrary, a decrease in smoking habit causes less incidence of cardiovascular disease. Indeed, the self-evident truth of such a concept is documented by the different number of smoker subjects and nonsmokers undergoing cardiovascular events provided by reports with similar data analyzed during different years [9–11].

An example is the number of deaths due to smoking reported to be of a different amount in the same Report when it is dated 1981 [9], 1983 [10], and 2004 [11], and this number reflects the trend of smoking. Nowadays, coronary heart disease [12] is responsible for the most deaths, and stroke ranks as the third leading cause of death, reaching in 2003, approximately 480,000 deaths for ischemic heart disease and 158,000 deaths for stroke. Moreover, a recent Report of the American Heart Association [13] estimates that 1.2 million of Americans suffer from a new or recurrent heart attack and approximately 700,000 individuals from new or recurrent stroke.

Smoking is one of the most important risk factors for those events which relate to atherosclerotic disease, a late but certain consequence of passive smoking exposure.

In the past, the number of people who died each year from smoking [4, 14], half of them before the age of 70 – an enormous human cost – was estimated in more than 3 million, and more than one third had cardiovascular events that often determine permanent disability of affected subjects. Today, more than 1 billion people smoke in the world and smoking habit varies widely with increased/decreased/ and again increased peaks [15].

This chapter will analyze the main clinical and pathological signs caused by passive smoking on cardiovascular system, and will describe the differences that exist between active smoking and passive smoking, as it can be see from the Table 4.1 about the type of pathology and localizations in the structures involved.

ATHEROSCLEROSIS

Atherosclerosis is a very complex entity that develops its alterations several years later from the isolated or more frequently, combined action of different triggering insults.

Several factors influence the course of the disease which is particularly related with the health status of people affected, genetic constitution, lifestyle, and exposure to a series of anatomical or functional injuries, some of them modifiable, on arterial wall.

There is a common evidence that people know the term atherosclerosis well, live together with it as if it is a habitual factor of life without considering the strongly negative consequences that atherosclerosis may cause. When the heavy complications due to atherosclerosis appear, then the individuals face up to the problem. Consequently, preventive measures against atherosclerosis are yet to be completely effective, although progresses to reduce the incidence of the disease begin to be seen because of a major knowledge of the risk factors.

Atherosclerotic lesions usually contain material of an inflammatory response associated with fibroproliferative manifestations [16–20]).

Passive smoking that is capable to cause endothelial dysfunction, which is considered the "door" of atherosclerosis [21] after both acute and chronic exposure, is a prominent factor for the development and progression of atherosclerotic pathology as there is evidence in several papers [8, 22– 24].

Pathologically, atherosclerosis is a dynamic process that causes the formation of an atherosclerotic plaque, often followed by complications as a result of a final pathway. Histologically, different steps characterize the degree of development of an atherosclerotic lesion. They are classified by the American Heart Association [25] in six types (Table 4.2.).

Table 4.2. Characteristics of the different types of atherosclerotic plaque

Atherosclerotic plaque	Type of Lesio
1. Type I	Accumulation of monocytes from the blood into the arterial intima across an intact endothelium.
2. Type II	Fatty streak: multifocal accumulation of lipid-foam cells beneath an intact endothelium.
3. Type III	Different size, but small, pools of extracellular lipid.
4. Type IV	Appearance of smooth muscle cells within the lesion beneath endothelium and formation of "lipid core" for coalescence of lipid pools.
5. Type V	Formation of a fibrous capsule containing the "lipid core" due to deposition of connective tissue (type Va), hard calcification (type Vb), and collagen, lipids and smoth muscle cells (type Vc).
6. Type VI	Complicated plaque with hemorrhage, thrombosis, rupture or embolization.

The dynamic of the atherosclerotic process is characterized by initial phases of cell migration [17, 26] beneath an intact endothelium. Monocytes reach the intima where undergo an activation and consequently conversion to macrophages. They catch lipids leading to formation of lipid-foam cells. These first stages are followed by multiple phases of accumulation and proliferation phenomena that determine fibrous capsule formation, lipid coalescence, calcification and smooth muscle cell disruption. These alterations are accompanied by heavy endothelial alterations.

Therefore, atherosclerotic plaque has three main components: 1. a cellular component with macrophages, smooth muscle cells, leukocytes and lipid-foam cells; 2. a fibrous matrix with connective tissue, collagen and elastic fibers; 3. a deposit of lipids coming from the intracellular and extracellular matrix, the amount of which varies widely and determines the structural characteristic of the plaque.

Observing the dynamic events of the atherosclerotic lesion, a significant fact appears. There is evidence that initial alterations occur with an intact endothelium. Normal endothelial function, as mentioned elsewhere, initially bars the progression of atherosclerotic injury, slowing its effects. On the contrary, if endothelial dysfunction occurs frequently, even in the case of transiently acute events, atherosclerotic plaque tends to form more quickly. Nowadays, there is undoubted evidence that both acute exposure and chronic exposure to passive smoking cause an early endothelial dysfunction [8, 23–24, 27–30], that can be transient but always reproducible in cases of acute exposure, either in healthy individuals or with a major severity, in individuals suffering from ischemic heart disease. Endothelial dysfunction strictly related to passive smoking triggers those changes which alter endothelium properties and accelerate atherosclerosis progression.

Since atherosclerosis is a term often used in a broad sense to indicate vascular alterations of a different type, it seems significant to clarify that passive smoking is particularly related to the development and progression of an atherosclerotic plaque rather than with other pathology of occlusive type, which may be also influenced negatively from smoking exposure. Moreover, when the alterations are due to a complication of atherosclerotic plaques as a result of passive smoking effects, usually the environmental exposure must last for a long time and be characterized by the presence of those factors listed in Table 1.5 of Chapter 1.

Atherosclerosis affects elastic and larger muscular arteries with a strong prevalence for those vessels which supply blood to the heart, brain, kidney and legs. All these organs are structures particularly altered by passive smoking exposure not only through a vascular mechanism of damage but also a mechanism due directly to toxic effects of smoking components.

Grossly, four types of alterations, which are exactly related to histologic aspect, may be seen: fatty streaks with or without yellow deposits of lipids which jut out vascular lumen; elevated fibrous plaques which may cause heavy narrowings in arterial diameter; plaques complicated by hemorrhagic phenomena or ulcerations which characterize the internal surface of intima of an irregularly pigmented ploughing; and then, calcified plaques are usually more stable and with less probability of embolization.

Complicated plaques are seen most frequently in populations who have a high incidence of fatal coronary artery disease [31], whereas superficial deposits of lipids may be found early in arteries of children aged six months and are a constant pattern after three years [32–33]. The real significance of this pattern is an object of findings since there are not unanimous opinions about its relationship with the development of future atherosclerosis.

The Figures 4.1 to 4.5 show the main characteristics of an atherosclerotic lesion. The wide spectrum of alterations that can be observed arises out of autopsy material of smokers and non-smokers who were examined in previous studies [34–36], and died from an ischemic cardiac or cerebral insult. All patients were older than 65 years, unless one young smoker woman who had 33 years and used oral contraception. She was suffering from angina and then, underwent a fatal acute myocardial infarction.

Generally, the atherosclerotic lesions found in smokers had a major severity than those observed in exposed nonsmokers. Exposed nonsmokers, however, showed a larger spectrum of alterations if compared with those subjects who died because of similar ischemic events and had not been exposed to environmental tobacco.

The age of the patients seemed to demonstrate either the prolonged time needed for the appearance of atherosclerotic complications or an earlier appearance if other risk factors were associated together in younger subjects.

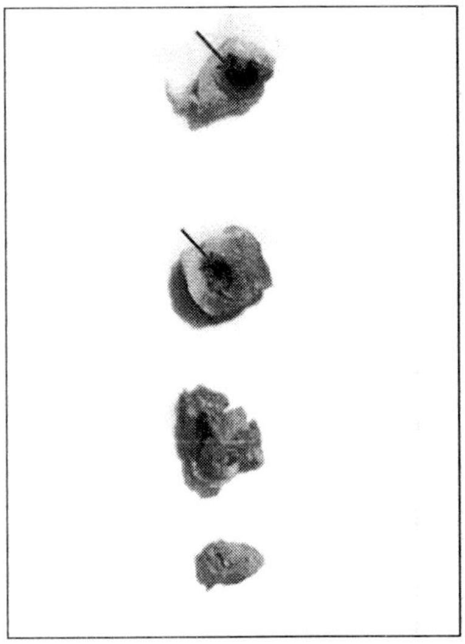

Figure 4.1.

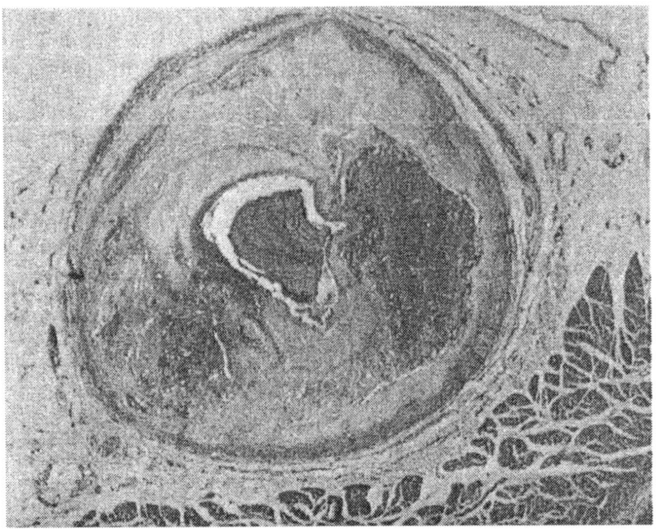

Figure 4.2.

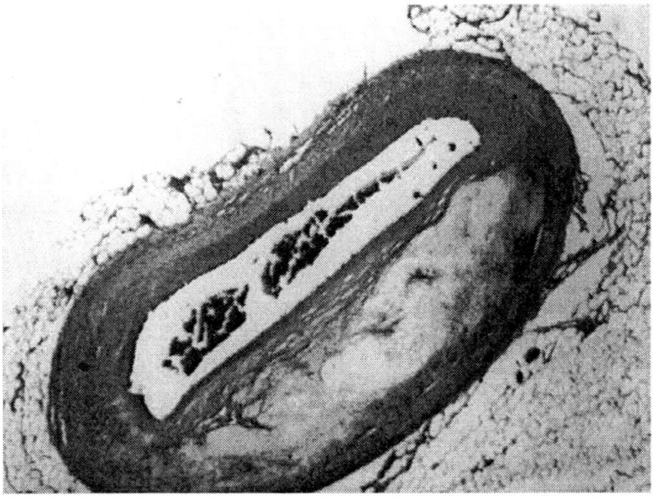

Figure 4.3.

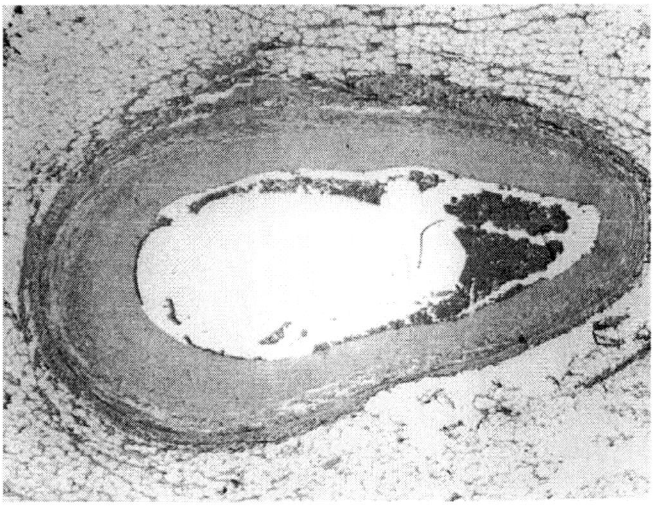

Figure 4.4.

Figure 4.1. to 4.4. Different alterations of coronary arteries due to atherosclerotic lesions of different degree and type. Figure 4.1. shows, macroscopically, the vessel lumen totally occluded by an old thrombus (red arrow); the thrombus narrows almost totally (95 percent of narrowing) vessel lumen on the coronary segment immediately below (red arrow). It also is showing the arterial wall with calcification. Histologically, the lumen of the vessel is occluded for about 95 percent by an old thrombus and arterial wall shows calcific deposits (Figure 4.2.). Figure 4.3. shows an eccentric narrowing with incomplete occlusion of the vessel lumen by an atherosclerotic plaque that is filled by lipid material and irregular calcium deposits. Figure 4.4. shows minimal atherosclerosis changes. One can see that the vessel lumen is almost totally pervious and irregular breaking of intima may be observed. Observing these different figures, there is a clear evidence of the "mosaic" of alterations that can characterize atherosclerotic disease.

Two main hypotheses try to explain the pathogenetic mechanisms of atherosclerosis: 1. A primary marked lipid role capable to initiate the disease, and 2. A repeated acute or chronic endothelial injury. They are probably acting together to cause the disease and in this way, explaining the multifactorial etiology of the disease.

The lipid hypothesis assigns primarily to disorders of lipid metabolism the mechanism triggering atherosclerosis. An elevated plasma LDL-Cholesterol concentration causes penetration of this substance into the arterial wall with its accumulation in smooth muscle cells and macrophages and lipid-foam cell formation. This phase is followed by all those processes described above which lead to fibrous cap formation as a final result.

Endothelial injury hypothesis, that is well related to Virchow triade (see Figure 3.8. of Chapter 3), postulates that different factors may induce endothelial dysfunction and consequently, adhesion of platelets to subendothelium, increased platelet aggregation, monocyte chemotaxis with release of a monocyte-derived growth factors that move smooth muscle cells from the media into the intima. Then, smooth muscle cells replicate and synthesize that fibrous material like connective tissue, collagen and proteoglycans that stimulates fibrous plaque formation.

There is no doubt that exposure to passive smoking can trigger those mechanisms of damage attributed to each of the hypotheses, responsible for atherosclerosis gerosis. In addition to endothelial damage, passive smoking accelerates the development of atherosclerosis because its negative effects on lipid metabolism [37]. Moreover, early studies suggest that there are specific agents derived from cigarette smoking able to damage the arterial wall [38] as well as presence of free radicals or different mutagens that activate smooth muscle cell proliferation [39].

About the appearance of clinical symptoms, three pathogenetic mechanisms have been postulated: firstly, occlusive thrombosis superimposed at a level of atherosclerotic plaque; secondly, plaque growing without thrombi and consequent production of a significant narrowing of the arterial lumen; thirdly, blood flow reduction due to external factors that precipitate an unstable vascular response. All these mechanisms are causing impairment in arterial blood flow but, may act only when atherosclerotic plaque is formed. Then, clinical symptoms usually occur several years later from the origin of the lesions.

In conclusion, there exist undoubted observations that a strong relationship between exposure to passive smoking and appearance of atherosclerosis cannot be denied.

Factors capable to induce atherosclerotic lesions are particularly the compounds of passive smoking, especially carbon monoxide and nicotine, that may induce endothelial dysfunction acutely and chronically either clinically or experimentally [8, 23 – 24, 30, 37, 40] as well as some characteristics related with the environment, type of exposure and health of exposed subjects [5].

Mechanisms of damage are known to be a repeated occurence of endothelial dysfunction, changes in blood coagulation cascade and platelet function [1, 23, 41–43], and lipid metabolism disorders [26. However, all those functional and biochemical factors can favor the development of thrombosis [1, 5, 17, 19, 37]. Current association of passive smoking exposure with other major cardiovascular risk factors accelerates the progression of atherosclerosis.

However, atherosclerotic plaque formation related with passive smoking exposure usually tends to appear late and pathologic events, particularly of ischemic type, are due to complications of an atherosclerotic lesion that more often is an irreversible structural alteration [3, 5].

Vascular structures particularly affected by atherosclerotic plaques are those of the heart, brain, and legs with possible recurrent clinical events that may determine a large spectrum of symptoms of ischemic heart disease, stroke, intermittent claudication or thrombotic gangrene. They often acutely demand intensive care and can also sometimes end the patient's life or cause a heavy and permanent disability for those subjects who are affected by these clinical alterations.

CORONARY HEART DISEASE

A direct relationship between a structural cardiovascular damage and exposure to passive smoking is not well demonstrated clinically in the sense that each exposure, differently to what occurs for the endothelial dysfunction, which is a common physiopathological basis for atherosclerosis development, causes a typical and constant alteration. However, a large series of epidemiological studies [44-56] that will be widely discussed in the next chapter of this book, support a strongly statistical evidence that chronic exposure to passive smoking is followed by a significant increase in coronary events, although these studies analyze the phenomenon, sometimes using different methodologies which often have no common approach to identify the environment characteristics, type and duration of passive smoking exposure, and people lifestyle.

On the contrary, experimentally acute exposure to passive smoking can cause impairment in exercise tolerance for both healthy individuals and individuals with a pre-existing myocardial infarction [57].

Coronary heart disease also recognizes a multifactorial etiology. Risk factors may play their effects isolately or with different combinations among themselves, inducing myocardial hypoxia. It may result from either a fall in oxygen transportation to the heart by coronary arteries or an increased demand in oxygen by cardiovascular system. Pathologically, a reduced availability in oxygen is a consequence of an impairment of coronary blood flow, less contact between cardiac fibers and intramyocardial coronary vessels, and reduced oxygen concentration of the blood. As previously described, two of these mechanisms, a decreased vascular coronary surface due to atherosclerotic narrowings with intraarterial lumen reduction and reduction in oxyhemoglobin concentration due to the effects of carbon monoxide, may be influenced by both active and passive smoking exposure.

Usually, coronary heart disease causes myocardial ischemia through an occlusion or narrowing of the lumen of one or plus coronary arteries because of a progression or complication of atherosclerotic plaques.

Whatever factor may induce coronary artery disease, the types of pathological patterns observed (Table 4.3.) are particularly angina pectoris, myocardial infarction, sudden death, arrhythmias and postischemic cardiomyopathy. Experimentally, there is evidence of a cardiomyopathy from smoking exposure [58–61]. Each of these events is characterized by typical structural alterations and clinical symptoms due to the disease but not to the factor capable to cause it, although from the analysis of the structural changes some features may be identified to be related to passive smoking. That is especially well inferred from the analysis of the type of alterations observed in experimental findings conducted on animals which had been exposed to passive smoking.

Table 4.3. Types of coronary heart disease and main mechanisms

Type of event	Main mechanism
1. Angina pectoris	Single or multiple coronary narrowings
2. Myocardial infarction	Myocardial muscle cell necrosis
3. Sudden death	Increased sympathetic stimulation
4. Arrhythmias (ventricular and atrial)	Increased sympathetic stimulation
5. Postischemic cardiomyopathy	Chronic and heavy hypoxia
6. Experimental cardiomyopathy	Smoking exposure

ANGINA PECTORIS, a clinical syndrome of ischemic heart disease with a typically retrosternal chest pain first described by Heberdeen [62], and is characterized by almost constant coronary atherosclerosis with coronary narrowings of different degree or total occlusions [63], isolated or multiple coronary vessel lumen, although other possible mechanisms as a coronary vasospasm [64], thrombosis and platelet aggregation [65] can interfere. Therefore, there is a strong relationship between cigarette smoking and angina, particularly stable angina, since the type of underlying coronary heart disease is coronary atherosclerosis with plaque progression or rupture, thrombosis and sometimes, functional vasospasm mediated by catecholamine release. Moreover, about 90% of the hearts of patients suffering from angina showed, at the postmortem examinations, different but severe degrees of coronary atherosclerosis [66–67].

Aronow [68] studied the effect of passive smoking on exercise-induced angina. Patients exposed to passive smoking had a larger increase in resting heart rate, systolic and diastolic blood pressure and venous carboxyhemoglobin and a greater reduction in heart rate and systolic blood pressure at angina with a significant reduction of exercise duration. Leone and coworkers [57] in their observations concerning both healthy individuals and individuals with a pre-existing myocardial infarction who were exposed acutely to passive smoking reached similar conclusions. Moreover, Meinert and coworkers [69] identified cigarette smoking as a factor of progression of coronary atherosclerosis in subjects with a pre-existing myocardial infarction. These observations will be discussed more widely in Chapter 9, where the characteristics of the experimental findings on harmful effects of environmental tobacco smoke are analyzed in detail.

Aristotle, a Greek philosopher, in his "Logic of Syllogism" [70], identified a form of reasoning in which, from two given or assumed propositions called major premise and minor premise having a common middle term, was deducted a third proposition, called logic conclusion, from which the middle term was absent and changed with the first term of the second premise. An example was: 1. All men are mortal; 2. Socrates is a man; 3. Therefore, Socrates is mortal. This assumed conclusion supported the logic of a phenomenon.

About the relationship existing between passive smoking and angina, the syllogism may be as follows: 1. Angina is due to coronary atherosclerosis; 2. Passive smoking causes coronary atherosclerosis; 3. Therefore, passive smoking causes angina (Table 4.4.).

From these observations, one cannot deny the close relationship between environmental tobacco smoke and angina, with this clinical symptom usually a manifestation of a coronary pathology characterized by the presence of either atherosclerosis or its complications.

Table 4.4. Aristotle' s syllogism applied to the relationship between passive smoking and angina

Syllogism propositions	Passive smoking/angina propositions
1. All men are mortal	1.Angina is due to coronary atherosclerosis
2. Socrates is a man	2. Passive smoking causes atherosclerosis
3. Socrates is mortal	3. Passive smoking causes angina

MYOCARDIAL INFARCTION is the most important manifestation of coronary heart disease and is the leading cause of morbidity and mortality in western countries.

Pathologically, it denotes the necrosis of a portion of myocardium due to insufficient acute blood supply.

Macroscopic and microscopic characteristics of myocardial infarction [71] have been well described for a long time and their aspect is common whatever the triggering cause, although, histologically, some little patterns may be observed in those subjects exposed to smoking [6, 73].

The main gross and microscopic changes of a myocardium affected by an infarction may be seen in Tables 4.5 and 4.6. Usually, pathological alterations may be documented after 6 to 12 hours from the onset of the disease with clinical symptoms often lacking in case of sudden coronary death. This fact sometimes causes great difficulties in establshing the true cause of death in a subject who does not yet show heart alterations at the autopsy. Not infrequent evidence of major coronary risk factors associated with pre-existing symptoms related to coronary involvement can lead one to suspect a possible acute myocardial infarction, since even histochemical procedures do not permit to assess a diagnosis before 6 hour time.

Table 4.5. Gross changes in acute myocardial infarction

Time of appearance	Characteristics
6/12 hours to 3 days	Myocardium pale and dry with red focal hemorrhagic areas.
4 to 8 days	Peripheral yellow zone extending into the dry myocardium.
8 to 12 days	Reduced myocardial wall thickness; yellow surface of infarct surronded by a red-purple depressed zone.
1° month	Red-purple material extends into infarct area.
2 to 3 months	Formation of a gray and firm scar at the infarct area.

Briefly, gross changes in acute myocardial infarction are the result of necrotic phenomena with a loss of myocardial structure of the affected area followed by processes of repair with formation of a firm and gray scar due to myocardial fibrosis.

Table 4.6. Microscopic changes in acute myocardial infarction

Time of appearance	Structural Characteristics
After 6 hours	Myocardial fibers swollen and acidophilic with loss of cross-striations, hyalinization, disappearance and pyknosis of nuclei.
First 5 days	Interstitial edema with capillary hyperemia; neutrophil infiltration and focal hemorrhage.
8 to 10 days	Dissolution of necrotic fibers and neutrophil infiltration into necrotic area; narrowings of granulation tissue at the margins of infarct area.
12 to 15 days	Appearance of collagen material.
3 to 4 weeks	ranulation tissue into the whole infarct area.
2 to 3 months	Great amount of collagen material.
3 month	Development of a firm fibrous scar.

Microscopic changes (Figure 4.5.) of a myocardial infarction follow a well defined pathway. Firstly, during two to three days from the onset of the disease, necrotic phenomena with polimorphonuclear infiltrates appear. Then, during the next 4 to 10 days, a granulation tissue into the infarct area tends to form, and finally, after two to three months, a firm scar completes the healing process. Therefore, neutrophil polymorphonuclears are the main characteristic living cells of the early stage that reach the dead zone of an infarction. However, these cells become too rapidly necrotic and their breaking really initiates all those repair processes which lead to fibrous scar formation, since a large amount of active enzymes and chemical substances deriving from polimorphonuclear degeneration clean up the infarct zone from necrotic material.

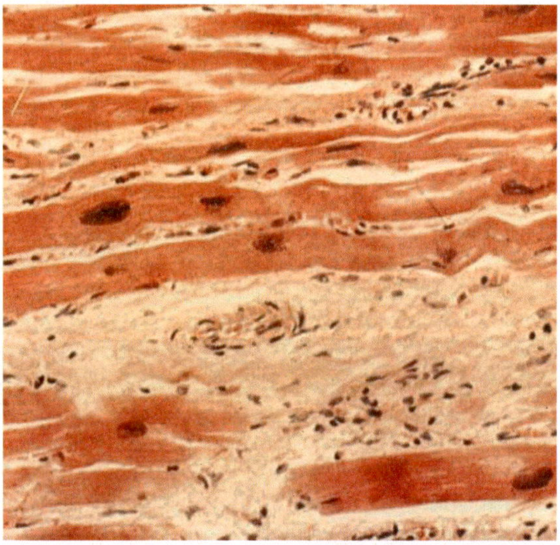

Figure 4.5. Myocardial infarction of 4 to 6 day-old. Several cardiocytes show focal or total lysis; many cardiocyte nuclei are intact, but there are cardiac fibers with disappearance of the nuclei; a central zone with polimorphonuclear infiltration and granulation tissue formation may also be seen.

Coronary arteries may show different degrees of narrowing, complete occlusions due to old thrombi, atherosclerothic plaque rupture with fresh thrombi superimposed and calcifications. However, myocardial infarctions with minimal or no coronary luminal reduction due to atherosclerosis at the necropsy have been described, and among these patients there were also smokers [72].

From these structurally basic alterations of a myocardial infarction, differences due to smoking exposure have been described [73].

Smoking exposure causes hemorrhagic microfocal infiltrates into the area affected by myocardial infarction with a major incidence. This occurence could be due to a direct effect of carbon monoxide on cardiac cells similarly to what has been demonstrated for the experimental cardiomyopathy from smoking. Moreover, in necropsy studies [6,73], the finding of more advanced narrowings of coronary artery characterized the smokers, particularly heavy smokers, when compared with nonsmokers passively exposed. These last subjects had however, a major incidence of coronary narrowings than those who never smoked, without passive smoking exposure. A major incidence of thickening of the small coronary vessels and calcifications affected particularly both smokers and nonsmokers who were exposed to environmental tobacco products. It is known that rise in intracellular calcium concentrations [74] with consequent calcification phenomena activates some enzyme chains that induce heavy cell injury until

cell death with complete loss of its function.

As one can see, passive smoking may cause myocardial infarction as a consequence of development, progression and complication of an atherosclerotic lesion. Moreover, structural alterations observed in both myocardial cells and coronary arteries are usually heavier than those in nonexposed smokers, never affected by a myocardial infarction.

SUDDEN DEATH [75] and ARRHYTHMIAS, particularly ventricular arrhythmias in patients with a pre-existing myocardial infarction after exposure to passive smoking [76], may also occur. However, a functional disorder due to increased catecholamine release, tends to cause these events, that will be discussed more in the next chapter concerning the functional disorders.

POSTISCHEMIC CARDIOMYOPATHY is a clinical event accompanied by heart failure with structural alterations usually characterized by degenerative lesions and fibrotic processes which are the result of a chronic repair following recurrent and acute hypoxic cardiovascular events. Multiple areas of microfocal fibrosis or confluent massive fibrosis impair cardiac function. A marked heart enlargement is a constant manifestation of this occurence.

EXPERIMENTAL CARDIOMYOPATHY has been described as a consequence of a direct effect of carbon monoxide toxicity on myocardium. Carbon monoxide effect may be potentiated by the reduced oxygen availability because of the higher affinity of carbon monoxide for hemoglobin. The structural features consist of focal areas of necrosis, particularly located in the subendocardium, perivascular infiltrates and typical punctate hemorrhages [77–78].

Cardiac involvement can appear early after exposure or more frequently, be a late manifestation. That strictly depends on either carbon monoxide concentration in the environment or duration of exposure. Ultrastructurally, mitochondria and intracellular respiratory chains are involved with heavy functional and metabolic alterations that lead, in time, to cardiac enlargement.

Cerebrovascular Disease

Cerebrovascular disease following passive smoking exposure may develop chronically as a result of repeated hypoxic insults or acutely as a stroke. Moreover, stroke can affect subjects with a pre-existing chronic cerebrovascular disease causing further impairment of brain function.

Cerebrovascular disease is a great problem of public health, being the third leading cause of death after coronary heart disease and all types of cancer [79]. Moreover, even if all risk factors of cerebrovascular disease and stroke, both ischemic stroke and hemorrhagic stroke, are removed, their incidence could be reduced to only a half [80]. Therefore, a large number of cerebrovascular events can be avoided and yet little knowledge about the real number of risk factors of cerebrovascular disease exists.

Hypertension, which is the factor in about 70% of stroke, increases the risk 6 fold; smoking could double the risk, and atrial fibrillation could cause strokes with an incidence similar to that of hypertension. Today, an effective control of these major risk factors tend to decrease the appearance of cerebrovascular disease.

Structurally, the alterations due to cerebrovascular disease may be classified into three types (Table 4.7.) according to the inducing mechanism: 1. Hypoxic changes, ischemia and infarction, which are all due to impairment in blood supply or oxygen availability; 2. Hemorrhagic lesions arising from to vessel rupture; 3.Combined synergism of the two previous events.

Table 4.7. Structural alterations in cerebrovascular disease

Type of cerebral alteration	Causative mechanism
1. Chronic hypoxic changes, ischemia, infarction	Blood supply impairment or poor oxygen availability.
2. Hemorrhagic lesions	Cerebral vessel rupture.
3. Combined type of alterations	Severe lesions in cerebral arteries from both mechanisms (1 + 2).

Cerebrovascular alterations are often associated with either vascular systemic changes, functional changes or anatomical changes. Intimal carotid thickness seems to play a strong role because of its strong relationship with cerebral arteries.

It has been well documented that passive smoking can induce progression of pre-existing atherosclerotic lesions as well as increase in thickness of carotid intima [81–82]. These manifestations can negatively influence the blood supply to cerebral areas. Moreover, a recent paper [83] analyzed the relationship between passive smoking and risk of acute stroke reaching the conclusion that there was a statistically significant increase in the risk of stroke in men and women who had been exposed to environmental tobacco smoke. The stroke risk increased further when those who had been exposed to passive smoking were excluded from the non-smoking reference group. Finally, authors underlined that studies investigating the adverse effects of smoking would be underestimated with regard to the risk of tobacco exposure since this parameter is not always taken into account. However, different opinions exist on the relationship between passive smoking and cerebrovascular disease. These differences will be again be discussed in Chapter 8 on the epidemiological studies.

Structurally, three main types of pathologic lesions of cerebrovascular system need to be discussed: ischemic cerebral infarction, hemorrhagic infarction, and chronic cerebral alterations, due to repeated insults from hypoxia. Cerebral metabolism is usually well balanced for what is concerning oxygen availability. Therefore, reduction in blood flow is an essential factor to induce cerebrovascular alterations.

Grossly, ischemic infarction follows three different phases with particular histologic patterns. During the first two days, affected area appears to be pale and swollen; then cerebral tissue becomes gelatinous and friable during the first week; finally tissue liquefies with formation of a cavity that can be surronded by a periphericaIly red-dark area.

Histologically, there is a change in cerebral white and gray structures with neuron alterations consisting of swelling, disintegration, and structural demyelinization. White blood cell infiltration and reletated phenomena of phagocytosis follow the initial phase during the first week; then, an evident infiltration in astrocytes floods affected area. These processes are so much more severe as the underlying atherosclerotic pathology. Passive smoking can impair the type and size of the cerebral lesion by three main mechanisms (Table 4.8.): 1. Causing a heavier degree of atherosclerosis; 2. Potentiating the effect of coagulation fibrinolysis cascade via thrombus formation; 3. Synergy with other major cardiovascular risk factors, particularly for those women using oral contraceptives. Among women, subarachnoid hemorrhage is more likely to occur in smokers than nonsmokers.

Table 4.8. Mechanisms by which passive smoking can impair a cerebral infarction

1. Relationship between passive smoking and degree of atherosclerotic lesions.
2. Thrombus formation by an activation of coagulation-fibrinolysis cascade.
3. Association with other major cardiovascular risk factors, particularly hypertension in men and oral contraceptives in women.

There is no evidence of a direct effect of passive smoking toxics to impair a cerebrovascular lesion. On the contrary, data seems to demonstrate few positive effects of smoking compounds on Alzheimer's disease [84]. However, other studies would seem to demonstrate that Alzheimer's disease is also influenced negatively by smoking [85–86]. Definitive conclusions with regard to this matter are far to be reached.

Cerebral hemorrhagic infarction is characterized by the same alterations of ischemic infarction but with the addition of phenomena of blood extravasation of different degree and amount and resorption that heavily influence the outcome of the lesion.

Finally, hypoxic alterations due to chronic and repeated insults of cerebral tissue without infarct area formation are characterized by different degrees of athrophy of both white and grey cerebral substance with a decrease in neuronal function and repair phenomena.

Table 4.9. summarizes the main gross and microscopic alterations observed in cerebral tissue as a consequence of the negative effects due to cerebrovascular pathology. It is evident that cerebrovascular alterations can have a different degree of extension with manifestations of isolated or multiple focal areas of damage, often confluent among themselves or massive areas of cerebral infarction that can be accompanied by atrophic phenomena of cerebral structure and compression of the brain.

Table 4.9. Main gross and microscopic alterations due to cerebrovascular events

Type	Gross changes	Microscopic changes
Ischemic infarction	1.Pale, swollen affected area	Neuronal swelling, disintegration, demyelinization.
	2. Gelatinous and friable tissue	White blood cell infiltration plus
	3. Cavity from cerebral liquefying	Astrocyte infiltration.
Hemorrhagic infarction	1 + 2 + 3 +	1 + 2 + 3 +
	4. Hemorrhagic zones into and at the margin of the infarct	Blood extravasation and resorption
Chronic hypoxia	1. Isolated or multiple areas	Cerebral atrophy and repair.

HYPERTENSION

A causal relationship between exposure to smoking and increase in blood pressure is not clearly demonstrated, although there are obsevations that seem to identify a transient increase in blood pressure while a subject is smoking a cigarette [1], as well as during acute exposure to passive smoking [1, 15, 29]. On the contrary, subjects exposed chronically to passive smoking could develop late a stable hypertension as a consequence of the progression of an atherosclerotic lesion. Moreover, endothelial dysfunction is strongly related to passive smoking exposure even in healthy people [8, 23–24]. It is assumed that endothelial dysfunction [87–88] has a strong association with hypertension. Endothelial dysfunction associated with essential hypertension is characterized by impaired nitric oxide (NO) availability attributable to oxidative stress production which causes NO breakdown [89].

Anatomical alterations specifically attributable to passive smoking exposure have not been identified as a direct consequence of this factor on blood pressure. Structural lesions documented in hypertensive patients exposed to environmental tobacco smoke are those of the hypertensive disease, its complications or disease causing hypertension. Therefore, atherosclerotic plaques with different degrees of narrowing, particularly in those vascular sites, are usually affected by atherosclerosis which may be found in hypertensive patients independently by their exposure to passive smoking, even if passive smoking could later cause hypertension.

PERIPHERAL ARTERIAL DISEASE

The relationship between smoking and peripheral arterial disease is well documented. Indeed, active smoking causes a typical pattern of arterial non-atherosclerotic occlusive disease that is known with the name of thromboangiitis obliterans or Buerger's disease [90].

Pathologic changes of Buerger's disease are characterized by segmental thrombosis, accompanied by acute and chronic inflammation of medium and small-size arteries, particularly of the legs and forearm with possible involvement of the adjacent veins and nerves [91].

The disease almost exclusively affects those men who smoke or have been heavy smokers during many years, even if they stop smoking. On the contrary, cessation of an early smoke can induce restoration and disappearance of the symptoms. An increased incidence of Buerger's disease has also been seen also in women and it could probably be related to their smoking habit.

Pathogenetically, a direct effect of tobacco smoke products has been postulated as well as hypersensitivity phenomena to some tobacco products without any direct toxic mechanism in Buerger's disease.

Clinically, claudication of a different degree is the most evident manifestation. Gangrene with amputation may conclude the spontaneous history of the disease, especially in continuing smokers.

Observations on the development of Buerger's disease people who have never smoked have been reported and they are probably related to breathing smoke, exhaled by others [92–93].

Anatomical changes of Buerger's disease deeply differ from those alterations that usually can be found in peripheral arteries of those subjects who did not suffer from thromboangiitis obliterans and were exposed to passive smoking exposure. Alterations for this group of subjects pathologically recognize a different mechanism linked to atherosclerotic disease.

Peripheral arterial occlusive disease particularly affects people who have a long history of smoking [94] in about 90% of cases. Autoptically, atherosclerosis has been observed particularly in aorta, lower limb arteries, carotids and coronary arteries which supply blood, as aforesaid, to those organs and tissues which negatively feel the effects of smoking.

It has been well established that five words could improve claudication [95] of leg arteries: "stop smoking and keep walking".

Biochemical connections [96] related to catecholamine levels have been also postulated as a pathogenetic factors for the development of peripheral arterial occlusive disease. Catecholamine effects and passive smoking will be discussed in the next chapter since functional disorders have been mainly documented as a consequence of an increased catecholamine release following passive smoking exposure.

Table 4.10 shows the main types of peripheral arterial occlusion as well as the main mechanisms that more often support vascular damage. These mechanisms may develop their effects either alone or by association among themselves, since inflammatory or infectious complications with impaired immunologic response [15], as a result of smoking exposure ,may occur and potentiate vascular damage.

Table 4.10. Main types of peripheral arterial occlusion

Disease	Characteristic
Atherosclerosis of the extremities	Atherosclerotic plaques complicated or not partially or totally occluding vessel lumen.
Thromboangiitis obliterans	Inflammatory occlusive vascular disorder.
Acute arterial occlusion	Sudden cessation of blood flow to extremity.
Atheroembolism	Embolization from a proximal atherosclerotic plaque with detrimental material.
Thoracic Outlet Compression Syndrome	Compression of the neurovascular bundle at the thoracic outlet.

It is worthwhile to be noted by Table 4.10, that all the above arterial occlusive syndromes can be the result of repeated insults due to passive smoking exposure, unless the last syndrome that recognizes cervical rib, scalenus muscle and clavicola first rib junction abnormalities without any underlying atherothrombotic lesions.

In conclusion, there is a clear evidence that passive smoking is a strong factor capable to induce peripheral artery occlusive pathology with pathological manifestations that can vary widely for morphology according to the degree of damage, extension, and pathogenetic mechanisms that produce the alterations.

Three main pathogenetic mechanisms, which are all related to passive smoking, may take part to determine vascular damage (Table 4.11.): 1. Atherosclerotic plaques; 2. Direct effect of toxic products contained into environmental tobacco smoke; 3. Hypersensitivity to tobacco smoke products, especially for thromboangiitis obliterans.

Table 4. 11. Mechanisms of damage from passive smoking in peripheral artery occlusion

1. Atherosclerotic plaque
2. Toxic effects of tobacco products
3. Allergic and inflammatory phenomena (thromboangiitis obliterans)

These mechanisms may be supported by frequent interference of functional factors particularly endothelial dysfunction and adrenergic stimulation that contribute actively to increase the level of occlusive lesions.

AORTIC ANEURYSMS

Every abnormal ballooning or localized dilatation of the arterial wall is an aneurysm. Aortic aneurysm is undoubtedly the most important form of aneurysm because the risk of bursting or clotting is higher than that of aneurysms of other peripheral arteries and often that causes catastrophic consequences for the affected patients.

There is a structural weakening of the arterial wall in aneurysms. It is usually a consequence of congenital defects, inflammation, trauma, localized or diffuse atherosclerotic processes or other degenerative pathology.

Atherosclerosis is the cause of about 70% of all aortic aneurysms [97], and a great majority of them affects abdominal aorta with renal artery involvement because of the major incidence of atherosclerotic lesions on abdominal aorta.

The relationship between smoking and aortic aneurysm has been well known for a long time [14, 98]. Studies have found a strong and, independent association between the two factors, concluding that smoking can cause aortic aneurysms. Observations identify that increased risk to develop an abdominal aortic aneurysm is found to be four to fivefold more frequent in active smokers than in nonsmokers [99]. Moreover, one study emphasizes the strong relationship existing between smoking and aortic aneurysm finding a very slow reduction in the risk of abdominal aortic aneurysm after smoking cessation [100].

Consistent data have demonstrated more and more that also passive smoking is also well related to the development of an aortic aneurysm [101 – 102].

Anatomical changes, which accompany the arterial wall when an aneurysm is developing, are different depending on the etiology and location of the disease. Changes in etiology have been found when past etiology was compared with etiology from today.

Blakemore and Voorhees [103] identified, in an autopsy study of the largest case-record of subjects, affected by aortic aneurysms, a clear prevailing of thoracic aneurysms from syphilis, while abdominal aneurysms recognized particularly an atherosclerotic etiology. However, aneurysm from syphilis had a major incidence from atherosclerosis.

Nowadays, with the almost total disappearance of syphilis, aortic aneurysm with atherosclerotic etiology is the most frequent occurence. It is followed by congenital aneurysms that, affect peripheral arteries, particularly arteries of the brain.

Grossly, a dilatation of the vessel differ in degree and extension in the basic pattern to diagnose an aneurysm.

Microscopically, the wall of an aneurysm is predominantly fibrous tissue with scarce traces of media into the vessel wall. Possible superimposed thrombi can produce emboli distally. The rupture of an aneurysm, especially of the aorta and cerebral arteries, is a dramatic and catastrophic event that often cause death of the patients. Rupture with massive hemorrhage usually occurs following an arterial wall breakdown or media dissecting and about 95% of affected people die within the first three days.

Table 4.12. summarizes the main gross and microscopic alterations that characterize an aortic aneurysm.

Table 4.12. Gross and microscopic changes in an aortic aneurysms

Gross changes:	Aortic dilatation of different extension and degree; Arterial wall weakening; Abdominal location(mainly) with frequent renal artery involvement.
Microscopic changes:	Fibrous tissue widely contained into the arterial wall; Thrombosis with possible distal embolization; rupture with massive hemorrhage; scarce traces of media.

Passive smoking and aortic aneurysms are more strictly linked by the development of atherosclerotic lesions, which often undergo complications, rather than by toxic effects of environmental tobacco smoke products.

References

[1] Glantz SA, Parmley WW: Passive smoking and heart disease. *JAMA.* 1995; 273: 1047 – 53.

[2] Leone A. The heart :a target organ for cigarette smoking. *J. Smoking-Related Dis.* 1992; 3: 197 – 201.

[3] Leone A. Cigarette smoking and health of the heart. *J. Roy. Soc. Health.* 1995; 115: 354 – 5.

[4] Wald NJ, Hackshaw AK. Cigarette smoking: an epidemiological overwiew. *British Medical Bulletin.* 1996; 52: 3 – 11.

[5] Leone A. Cardiovascular damage from smoking: a fact or belief? *Int. J. Cardiol.* 1993; 38: 113 – 7.

[6] Auerbach O, Carter HW, Garfinkel L, Hammond EC. Cigarette smoking and coronary heart disease, a macroscopic and microscopic study. *Chest.* 1976; 70: 697 – 705.

[7] Penn A, Chen LC, Snyder CA. Inhalation of steady-state sidestream smoke from cigarettes promotes arteriosclerotic plaque development. *Circulation.* 1994; 90: 1363 – 7.

[8] Giannini D, Leone A, Nuti M, Strata G, Balbarini A, Mariani M. Indoor passive smoking impairs endothelial function. *European Heart Journal.* 2001; 22: 128A.

[9] US Department of Health and Human Services. The health consequences of involuntary smoking. A Report of the Surgeon General. Rockville, MD: Public Health Service, Center for Disease Control, Center for Health Promotion and Education, Office on Smoking and Health, 1981; *DHHS Publication.* n° (CDC) 87 – 8398.

[10] US Department of Health, Education, and Welfare: The health consequences of smoking: a Report of the Surgeon General. Cardiovascular Disease. Rockville, MD: US Department of Health and Human Services, Public Health Service Office of Smoking and Health. *DHHS Publication.* n° (PHS) 84- 50204, 1983.

[11] US Department of Health and Human Services . The health consequences of smoking: A Report of the Surgeon General. Atlanta: US Department of Health and Human Services, Centers for Disease Control and Prevention, National Center for Chronic Disease Prevention and Health Promotion, Office on Smoking and Health, 2004.

[12] Hoyert DL, Heron M, Murphy SL, Kungo H-C. Deaths: final data for 2003, January 19, 2006;http://www.cdc.gov/nchs/products/pubs/pubd/hestats/finaldeaths03/finaldeaths03.htm; accessed: February 14, 2006.

[13] American Heart Association. Heart and Stroke Statistics – 2005 Update. Dallas: American Heart Association, 2005.

[14] Peto R, Lopez AD, Boreham J, Thun M, Heath C. Mortality from smoking in developed countries: 1950 – 2000. Oxford: Oxford University Press 1994.

[15] Leone A. Biochemical markers of cardiovascular damage from tobacco smoke. *Curr. Pharm. Design.* 2005; 11: 2199 – 2208.

[16] Stary HC. Macrophages, macrophage foam cells, and eccentric intimal thickening in the coronary arteries of young children. *Atherosclerosis.* 1987; 64: 91 – 108.

[17] Ross R. The pathogenesis of atherosclerosis: A perspective for the 1990s. *Nature.* 1993; 362: 801 – 9.

[18] Wissler RW, Hiltscher L, Oinuma T, for PDAY Research Group. The lesions of atherosclerosis in the young: From fatty streaks to intermediate lesions. In: Fuster V, Ross R, Topol EJ eds. *Atherosclerosis and Coronary Artery Disease*. Philadelphia, USA, Lippincot- Raven 1996; 475 – 89.

[19] Ross R. The pathogenesis of atherosclerosis- un update. *N. Engl. J. Med.* 1986; 314: 488 – 500.

[20] McGill HC Jr. Atherosclerosis: Problems in pathgenesis. *Atheroscler. Rev.* 1977; 2: 27 – 65.

[21] Desideri G, Ferri C. Endothelial activation. Sliding door to atherosclerosis. *Curr. Pharm. Design.* 2005; 11: 2163 – 75.

[22] Werner RM, Pearson TA. What is so passive about passive smoking? Secondhand smoke as a cause of atherosclerotic disease. *JAMA.* 1998; 279: 157 – 8.

[23] Davis J, Shelton L, Watanabe I, Arnold J. Passive smoking affects endothelium and platelets. *Arch. Intern. Med.* 1989; 149: 386 – 9.

[24] Celermajer DS, Sorensen KE, Georgakopoulos D. Cigarette smoking is associated with dose-related and potentially reversible impairment of endothelium-dependent dilation in healthy young adults. *Circulation.* 1993; 88: 2149 – 55.

[25] American Heart Association. A definition of advanced types of atherosclerotic lesions and a histological classification of atherosclerosis: A report from the Committee on Vascular Lesions of the Council of Atherosclerosis. *Circulation.* 1995; 92: 1355 – 74.

[26] Faggiotto A, Ross R, Harker L. Studies of hypercholesterolemia in the non-human primate: I. Changes that lead to fatty streak formation. *Arteriosclerosis.* 1984; 4: 323 – 40.

[27] Sumida H, Watanabe H, Kugiyama K, Ohgushi M, Matsumura T, Yasue H. Does passive smoking impair endothelium-dependent coronary artery dilation in women? *J. Am. Coll. Cardiol.* 1998; 31: 811 – 5.

[28] Powell JT. Vascular damage from smoking: disease mechanisms at the arterial wall. *Vasc. Med.* 1998; 3: 21 – 8.

[29] Leone A. Relationship between cigarette smoking and other coronary risk factors in atherosclerosis: risk of cardiovascular disease and preventive measures. *Curr. Pharm. Design.* 2003; 9: 2417 – 23.

[30] Deanfield J. Passive smoking and early arterial damage. *European Heart Journal.* 1996; 17: 645 – 6.

[31] Gore I, Robertson WB, Hirst AE, Hadley GG, Koseki Y. Geographic differences in the severity of aortic and coronary atherosclerosis: the U.S., Jamaica, W.L., South India, and Japan. *Amer. J. Path.* 1960; 36: 559 – 74.

[32] Zinserling WD. Untersuchungen uber atherosclerose. I. Uber die aortenverfettung bei kindern. *Virchow Arch. Path. Anat.* 1925; 225: 677 – 705.

[33] Holman RL, McGill HC jr, Strong JP, Geer JC. The natural history of atherosclerosis. The early aortic lesions as seen in New Orleans in the middle of the 20th century. *Am. J. Path.* 1958; 34: 209 – 35.

[34] Leone A, Lopez M. Role du tabac et de la contraception orale dans l'infarctus du myocarde de la femme. Description d'un cas. *Pathologica.* 1984 ; 76 : 493 – 8.

[35] Leone A, Lopez M. Oral contraception, ovarian disorders and tobacco in myocardial infarction of woman. *Pathologica.* 1986; 78: 237 – 42.

[36] Leone A. Cigarette smoking and cardiovascular damage: analytic review of the subject. *Singapore Med. J.* 1994; 35: 492 – 4.
[37] Barnoya J, Glantz SA. Cardiovascular effects of secondhand smoke: nearly as large as smoking. *Circulation.* 2005; 111:2684 – 98.
[38] Becker CG, Dubin T, Wiedemann HP. Hypersensitivity to tobacco antigen. *Proc. Natl. Acad. Sci. USA.* 1976; 73: 1712 – 6.
[39] Stafford RS, Becker CG. Cigarette smoking and atherosclerosis. In: Fuster V, Ross R, Topol EJ eds. *Atherosclerosis and Coronary Artery Disease.* Lippincott-Raven, Philadelphia, USA, 1996; 303 – 25.
[40] Mullick AE, McDonald JM, Melkonian G, Talbot P, Pinkerton KE, Rutledge JC. Reactive carbonyls from tobacco smoke increase arterial endothelial layer injury. *Am. J. Physiol. Heart Circ. Physiol.* 2002; 283: H591 – 7.
[41] Law MR, Morris JK, Wald NJ. Environmental tobacco smoke exposure and ischemic heart disease: an evaluation of the evidence. *BMJ.* 1997; 315: 973 – 80.
[42] Ambrose JA, Barua RS. The pathophysiology of cigarette smoking and cardiovascular disease: an update. *J. Am. Coll. Cardiol.* 2004; 43: 1731 – 7.
[43] Davis JW, Hartman CR, Lewis HD Jr., Shelton L, Eigenberg DA, Hassanein KM, Hignite CE, Ruttinger HA. Cigarette smoking-induced enhancement of platelet function: lack of prevention by aspirin in men with coronary artery disease. *J. Lab. Clin. Med.* 1985; 105: 479 – 83.
[44] Sherman CB. Health effects of cigarette smoking. *Clin. Chest. Med.* 1991; 12: 643 – 58.
[45] Thun M, Henley J, Apicella L. Epidemiologic studies of fatal and nonfatal cardiovascular disease and ETS exposure from spousal smoking. *Environ Health Perspect.* 1999; 107S: 841 – 6.
[46] Wells AJ. Passive smoking as a cause of heart disease. *J. Am. Coll. Cardiol.* 1994; 24: 546 – 54.
[47] Doll R, Peto R. Mortality in relation to smoking: 20 years' observations on male British doctors. *BMJ.* 1976; 2: 1525 – 36.
[48] Steenland K. Passive smoking and the risk of the heart disease. *JAMA.* 1992; 267: 94 – 9.
[49] Kawachi I, Colditz GA, Speizer FE, Manson JE, Stampfer MG, Willet W, Hennekens C. A prospective study of passive smoking and coronary heart disease. *Circulation.* 1997; 95: 2374 – 9.
[50] Helsing K, Sandler D, Comstock G, Chee E. Heart disease mortality in nonsmokers living with smokers. *Am. J. Epidemiol.* 1988; 127: 915 – 22.
[51] Hole D, Gillis C, Chopra C, Hawthorne VM. Passive smoking and cardiorespiratory health in a general population in the west of Scotland. *BMJ.* 1989; 299: 423 – 7.
[52] LeVois ME, Layard MW. Publication bias in the environmental tobacco smoke/coronary heart disease epidemiologic literature. *Regul. Toxicol. Pharmacol.* 1995; 21: 184 – 91.
[53] Steenland K, Thun M, Lally C, Heath C Jr. Environmental tobacco smoke and coronary heart disease in the American Cancer Society CPS-II cohort. *Circulation.* 1996; 94: 622 – 8.
[54] Dobson AJ, Alexander HM, Heller RF, Lloyd DM. Passive smoking and the risk of heart attack or coronary death . *Med. J. Aust.* 1991; 154: 793 – 7.

[55] Muscat JE, Wynder EL. Exposure to environmental tobacco smoke and the risk of heart attack. *Int. J. Epidemiol.* 1995; 24: 715 – 9.

[56] He Y, Lam TH, Li LS, Du RY, Jia GL, Huang JY, Zheng JS. Passive smoking at work as a risk factor for coronary heart disease in Chinese women who have never smoked. *BMJ.* 1994; 308: 380 – 4.

[57] Leone A, Mori L, Bertanelli F, Fabiano P, Filippelli M. Indoor passive smoking: its effect on cardiac performance. *Int. J. Cardiol.* 1991; 33: 247 – 52.

[58] Lough J. Cardiomyopathy produced by cigarette smoke. Ultrastructural observations in guinea pigs. *Arch. Pathol. Lab. Med.* 1978; 102: 377 – 80.

[59] Gvozdjakova A, Bada V, Sany L, Kucharska J, Kruty F, Bozek P, Trstansky L, Gvozdjak J. Smoke cardiomyopathy: disturbance of oxidative processes in myocardial mitochondria. *Cardiovascular Research.* 1984; 18: 229 – 32.

[60] Kjeldsen K, Thomsen HK, Astrup P. Effects of carbon monoxide on myocardium. Ultrastructural changes in rabbits after moderate, chronic exposure. *Circ. Res.* 1974; 34: 339 – 48.

[61] Gvozdjakova A, Kucharska J, Gvozdjak J. Effect of smoking on the oxidative processes of cardiomyocytes. *Cardiology.* 1992; 1992: 81 – 4.

[62] Heberdeen W. Angina Pectoris. Medical Transactions of the Royal College of Physicians 1772.

[63] Blumgart HL, Schlesinger MJ, Davis D. Studies on the relation of the clinical manifestations of angina pectoris, coronary thrombosis, and myocardial infarction to the pathologic findings. *Amer. Heart J.* 1940; 19: 1 – 91.

[64] Maseri A, Severi S, De Nes M, L'Abbate A, Chierchia S, Marzilli M, Ballestra AM, Parodi O, Biagini A, Distante A. Variant angina: one aspect of a continuous spectrum of vasospastic myocardial ischemia. Pathogenetic mechanisms, estimated incidence, clinical and coronarographic findings in 138 patients. *Am. J. Cardiol.* 1978; 42: 1019 – 35.

[65] Folts JD, Crowell EB, Rowe G. Platelet aggregation in partially obstructed vessels and its elimination with aspirin. *Circulation.* 1976; 54: 365 – 70.

[66] Blumgart HL, Pitt B, Zoll PM, Freiman DG. Anatomic factors influencing the locations of coronary occlusions and development of collateral coronary circulation. In:*The Etiology of myocardial infarction,* James TN and Keys JW eds. Little, Brown, Boston 1963; 327 – 37.

[67] Blumgart HL, Zoll PM, Wessler S. Angina pectoris; clinical pathologic study of 177 cases. *Trans. Ass. Amer. Physicians.* 1950; 63: 262 – 7.

[68] Aronow WS. Effect of passive smoking on angina pectoris. *N. Engl. J. Med.* 1978; 299: 21 – 4.

[69] Meinert CL, Forman S, Jacobs DR, Stamler J. Cigarette smoking as a risk factor in men with a prior history of myocardial infarction. *J. Chronic. Dis.* 1979; 32: 415 – 25.

[70] Russel B. The Logic of Aristotle. In: *Russel B ed. History of western philosophy and its connection with political and social circumstances from the earliest time to the present day.* Longanesi Publishing, Milan, Italy, 1966; 271 – 80.

[71] Mallory GK, White PD, Salcedo-Salgar J. The speed of healing of myocardial infarction. A study of the pathologic anatomy in seventy-two cases. *Amer. Heart J.* 1939; 18: 647 – 71.

[72] Eliot RS, Baroldi G, Leone A. Necropsy studies in myocardial infarction with minimal or no coronary luminal reduction due to atherosclerosis. *Circulation.* 1974; 49: 1127 – 31.

[73] Leone A, Bertanelli F, Mori L, Fabiano P, Battaglia A. Features of ischaemic cardiac pathology from cigarette smoking. *J. Smoking-Related Dis.* 1994; 5: 109 – 14.

[74] Trump BJ, Berezesky I. The reactions of cells to lethal injury: oncosis and necrosis- the role of calcium. In Lockshin RA et al. Eds: *When cells die – A comprehensive evaluation of apoptosis and programmed cell death.* Wiley-Liss, New York 1998; 57 – 96.

[75] Health or Smoking. Follow-up report of the Royal College of Physicians . Pitman Publishing, London 1983.

[76] Leone A, Bertanelli F, Mori L, Fabiano P, Bertoncini G. Ventricular arrhythmias by passive smoke in patients with pre-existing myocardial infarction. *J. Am. Coll. Cardiol.* 1992; 3: 256A.

[77] McMeekin JD, Finegan BA. Reversible myocardial dysfunction following carbon monoxide poisoning. *Can. J. Cardiol.* 1987; 3: 118 – 121.

[78] Leone A, Tagliagambe A. Long-term prognosis of infarcted smokers: is it affected by smoking cessation? In: Aoki M, Hisamichi S, Tominaga S eds. *Smoking and Health.* 1987. Elsevier/North Holland, Amsterdam, 1988; 723 – 6.

[79] National Center for Health Statistics. Monthly vital statistics report. US Department of Health and Human Services, Public Health Service, Office of Health Research, Statistics, and Technology, National Center for Health Statistics. *DHHS Publication.* n° (PHS) 80 – 1120; 1980; 29 Suppl 1.

[80] Hachinski V. Stroke prevention. In: Aquino AV, Piedad FF, Sulit YQM, 23rd Congress of International Society of Internal Medicine; Monduzzi International Proceedings Division, Bologna, Italy, 1996; 257 – 61.

[81] Howard J, Burke GL, Szklo M, Tell GS, Eckfeldt J, Evans G, Heiss G. Active and passive smoking are associated with increased carotid wall thickness. *Arch. Intern. Med.* 1994; 154: 1277 – 82.

[82] Howard J, Wagenknecht LE, Burke GL, Diez-Roux A, Evans GW, McGovern P, Nieto J, Tell GS, for the ARIC Investigators. Cigarette smoking and progression of atherosclerosis: The atherosclerosis risk in communities (ARIC) study. *JAMA.* 1998; 279: 119 – 24.

[83] Bonita R, Duncan J, Truelsen T, Jackson RT, Beaglehole R. Passive smoking as well as active smoking increases the risk of acute stroke. *Tob. Control.* 1999; 8: 156 – 60.

[84] News- Medical Net. Cigarette smoking may lower rates of neurodegenerative diseases like Parkinson's and Alzheimer's. March 15, 2004.

[85] Butler R. Current cigarette smoking was associated with a higher risk of Alzheimer's disease. *Evid. Based Ment. Health.* 1999; 2: 126.

[86] Merchant C, Tang MX, Albert S, Manly J, Stern Y, Mayeux R. The influence of smoking on the risk of Alzheimer's disease. *Neurology.* 1999; 52: 1408 – 12.

[87] Panza JA, Quyyumi AA, Brush JE Jr, Epstein SE. Abnormal endothelium-dependent vascular relaxation in patients with essential hypertension. *N. Engl. J. Med.* 1990; 323: 22 – 7.

[88] John S, Schmieder RE. Impaired endothelial function in arterial hypertension and hypercholesterolemia: potential mechanisms and differences. *J. Hypertens.* 2000; 18: 363 – 74.

[89] Taddei S, Virdis A, Ghiadoni L, Magagna A, Salvetti A. Vitamin C improves endothelium-dependent vasodilation by restoring nitric oxide activity in essential hypertension. *Circulation.* 1998; 97: 2222 – 9.

[90] Buerger L. Thrombo-angiitis obliterans: a study of the vascular lesions leading to presenile spontaneous gangrene. *Am. J. Med. Sci.* 1908; 136: 567 – 80.

[91] Joyce JW. Buerger's disease (thromboangiitis obliterans). *Rheum. Dis. clin. North Am.* 1990; 16: 463 – 70.

[92] Young C, Beynon H, Haskard D. Buerger's disease (thromboangiitis obliterans): a reversible cause of upper limb digital infarcts. *Rheumatology.* 2000; 39: 442 – 3.

[93] Lambotte O, Chazerain P, Vinciguerra C, Meyer O, Ziza JM. Thromboangiitis obliterans with inaugural rheumatic manifestations. A report of three cases. *Rev. Rhum. Engl. Ed.* 1997; 64: 334 – 8.

[94] Fowkes FGR. Aetiology of peripheral atherosclerosis. Smoking seems especially important. *BMJ.* 1989; 298: 405 – 6.

[95] Housley E. Treating claudication in five words. *BMJ.* 1988: 296: 1483 – 4.

[96] Lassila R, Laustiola KE. Cigarette smoking and peripheral arterial occlusive disease – evidence for adrenergic connections. *J. Smoking-Related Dis.* 1992; 3: 217 – 23.

[97] Halpert B, Willms RK. Aneurysms of the aorta. An analysis of 249 necropsies. *Arch. Path.* 1962; 74: 163 – 8.

[98] Hammond EC, Garfinkel L. Coronary heart disease, stroke and aortic aneurysm. *Arch. Environ. Health.* 1969; 19: 167 – 82.

[99] Doll R, Peto R, Wheatley K, Gray R, Sutherland I. Mortality in relation to smoking: 40 years' observations on male British doctors. *BMJ.* 1994; 309: 901 – 11.

[100] Wilmink TB, Quick CR, , Day NE. The association between cigarette smoking and abdominal aortic aneurysm. *J. Vasc. Surgery.* 1999; 30: 1099 – 105.

[101] Vardulaki KA, Walker NM, Day NE, Duffy SW, Ashton HA, Scott RAP. Quantifying the risk of hypertension, age, sex, and smoking in patients with abdominal aortic aneurysm. *Br. J. Surgery.* 2000; 87: 195 – 200.

[102] Ernst CB. Current concepts: abdominal aortic aneurysm: *N. Engl. J. Med.* 1993; 328: 1167 – 72.

[103] Blakemore AH, Voorhees AB Jr. Aneurysm of the aorta. A review of 365 cases. *Angiology.* 1954; 5: 209 – 31.

Chapter 5

Functional Disorders of Cardiovascular System

Abstract

Functional disorders of cardiovascular system from exposure to passive smoking are due to increased catecholamine release and endothelial dysfunction that, physio-pathologically, are strongly related.

Nicotine, but also carbon monoxide, favor the appearance of those phenomena attributable to adrenergic system stimulation consisting, particularly, of increased hemodynamic function, increased heart rate with loss of heart rate variability, increase in systolic blood pressure in presence of epineprine release, and increase in both systolic and diastolic blood pressure in presence of norepinephrine.

Endothelial dysfunction, currently assessed by brachial artery ultrasonography, appears to be an effect of reduced availability of endothelial vasodilator chemicals – nitric oxide – and concomitant increase in endothelin, a strong vasoconstrictor. A direct chemical injury determined particularly by nicotine, its metabolites, and carbon monoxide occurs since a large majority of other passive smoking compounds has mainly carcinogenic rather than cardiovascular effects.

A partial restoration of physiological functions of those structures that are altered characterizes passive smoking exposure cessation, particularly with regard to endothelial dysfunction. However, functional disorders from passive smoking usually are the "door" of heavy structural alterations that conclude the course of chronic exposure.

Keywords: Functional disorder (s), nicotine, carbon monoxide, catecholamine release, epinephrine, norepinephrine, dopamine, sympathetic nervous ending(s), adrenal gland, chromaffin tissue, heart rate, hemodynamic changes, systolic blood pressure, diastolic blood pressure, endothelium, endothelium-dependent vasodilation, nitric oxide, endothelin, circulating progenitor cell(s), brachial artery ultrasonography.

Functional disorders of cardiovascular system are the clearest evidence of damage from passive smoking in exposed individuals for three main reasons: 1. Early and almost constant appearance, although most often transiently, during and immediately after smoking exposure; 2. Easy assessment by simple diagnostic procedures, particularly vascular echography; 3. Reproducibility of the results after acute exposure of the subjects in the same experimental conditions.

Findings demonstrate undoubtedly the truthfulness of the above statements [1 – 3]. Bare necessities to interpret correctly the significance of a functional disorder are establishing what it is, what it causes, and how to recognize the types of its response.

WHAT IS A FUNCTIONAL DISORDER ?

A functional disorder consists of an abnormal response, usually transient and accompanied by physical symptoms, of body structures with a proper and constant function following a stimulus that tends to change the normal level of response of a psysiologically stimulated structure. Stimulus can be characterized by a higher threshold or a lower threshold with regard to the function of the structure and then it can induce overstimulation or a response of a level lower than that usually produced. Applied stimuli can be of different types, biological, biochemical, toxicological, pathological, and of other types. However, they have the characteristic to always cause a similar response when two conditions are satisfied: 1. Each applied stimulus must have the same level of threshold, and 2. Functionally, the structure that undergoes stimulus must be in the same baseline condition in which the previous stimulus of which we want to reproduce the effects was applied.

No stimulus causes a functional response localized to a single structure of the body. That is due to the fact that usually, its action affects receptors which are spread on different sites. However, a more selective response belongs to those structures mainly provided in a great amount by specific receptors towards the specific stimulating substance. There is evidence that such a condition regulates the relationship between passive smoking and some metabolites, particularly catecholamines and those chemicals which may involve negatively the endothelial function.

It has to be emphasized that the response to functional stimuli is a functional response, but not necessarily the stimulus, which can be different in type, intensity, duration, and frequency of action, inducing the same effects. According to these characteristics, the functional response that stimulus induces can vary its properties (Figure 5.1.), as well as type of restoration.

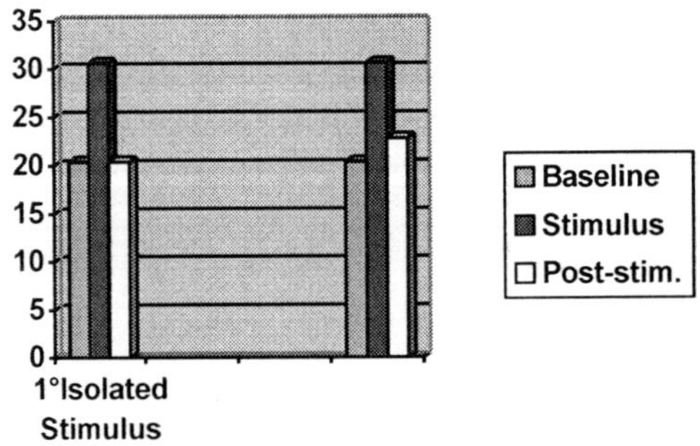

Figure 5.1. Functional response to stimuli. Isolated stimulus induces an amount in structure response followed by a return to a baseline function. On the contrary, repeated stimuli determine, in time, an increased level of baseline function.

An isolated stimulus that exceeds the baseline response threshold of the structure induces transiently functional symptoms that enhance the function while it is acting; immediately after the end of the stimulus, a mild decrease in baseline function can be observed; then, a rapid restoration of baseline function follows the previous phase.

Moreover, if the stimulus stresses a response of the structure most frequently as applying time or by a threshold level always higher than that of baseline response, a stable post-stimulus hyperfunction of structure can be induced. Consequently, the baseline response will regulate itself at a permanent more elevated level that can determine the initial appearance of anatomical alterations.

Different effects are caused by a stimulus when its threshold level is lower than that of the baseline response. Stimulated structure ignores the intensity of the stimulus when it is isolated. On the contrary, when the stimulus with a lower threshold influences most frequently the structure, the baseline response can undergo an impairment regulating its level to a lower step than previously.

In both cases, however, functional response changes in time, its characteristic leading to the appearance of alterations which can usually modify the the level of initial baseline function.

Occurences like those may characterize cardiovascular response to a stimulus induced by toxic chemicals of passive smoking.

The purpose of this chapter is to describe biochemical and physiological properties of catecholamines as well as endothelium and then analyze cardiovascular response to these parameters after environmental tobacco smoke exposure.

Moreover, according to what has been described above, it has to be emphasized that passive smoking influences functionally cardiovascular system by an overstimulation of catecholamine release and some endothelial metabolites that impair cardiovascular function. A reduced function and concentration for those endothelial chemicals that usually protect endothelial integrity is also induced by passive smoking.

Catecholamine Biochemistry and Physiology

Two chemical compounds have been isolated from adrenal medullary extracts, epinephrine and norepinephrine. They are stored in separate cells of the medulla and are relaxed by intercurrent metabolic events, accelerated metabolism, stimuli of different types. The release of catecholamines from the adrenal medulla is influenced by acetylcholine in the presence of calcium ions. This is the final step of a complex series of changes that involve autonomic system, endocrine glands and some biometabolites that separately or all together may be influenced by passive smoking exposure.

Catecholamines [4] are also stored in a large chromaffin tissue that develops in several structures of the body: sympathetic ganglions, localized along the course of abdominal aorta, and all ganglionic sites that accompany sympathetic nerve endings. Intratissutal catecholamines are produced in several organs and the third natural catecholamine, dopamine, is also stored in a peripheral dopaminergic system not yet identified. Usually, catecholamines exert their activity where they are released or all around.

Epinephrine, norepinephrine and dopamine are neurotransmitters in the central nervous system. Outside this structure, the activity of the catecholamines differ. Epinephrine is a hormone of adrenal medulla with a prompt availability according to many requirements, mostly linked to stress or acute stimuli capable to realize stressing positions. On the contrary, norepinephrine acts primarily as a neurotransmitter of sympathetic postganglionic neurons; it is related to preganglionic neuron acetylcholine to regulate sympathetic activity. The third catecholamine, dopamine, has an unclear role and probably acts particularly as a neurotransmitter with a primary activity on cerebral structures.

Biochemically, catecholamines derive from the amino acid tyrosine by a complex process of hydroxylation, decarboxylation, and again, hydroxylation. Figure 5.2. shows the main metabolic pathways to synthesize catecholamines.

The main pathways to synthesize the hormones occur in different structures like liver, kidney, brain, but particularly the adrenal gland. A complex mechanism of feed-back that involves many structures as adrenoreceptors, peripheral tissues, metabolic and functional cell responses regulates catecholamine biosynthesis and release. Catecholamines lead their activity, particularly to those structures like cardiovascular system, which feel like early stressing stimuli. They require a major availability of either those metabolites capable to accelerate cardiac and vascular function or oxygen. According to the different types of responses that catecholamines determine, an acute stimulation of cardiovascular system initiated by epinephrine could be prolonged by increased release and stimulation due to norepinephrine. Therefore, it is sometimes hard to establish what it is due to a hormone and what to the other.

Phenylananine

↓ **Hydroxylation (liver)**

Tyrosine

↓ **Oxidation (adrenal gland)**

3,4-dihydroxyphenylalanine-dopa-

↓ **Decarboxylation (kidney, liver, adrenal gland)**

3,4-dihydroxyphenylethylamine- hydroxytyramine-

↓ **Hydroxylation**

Norepinephrine

↓ **Methylation (adrenal gland)**

Epinephrine

Figure 5.2. Main metabolic pathways for catecholamine biosynthesis.

Chemical formula of epinephrine and norepinephrine is as follows:

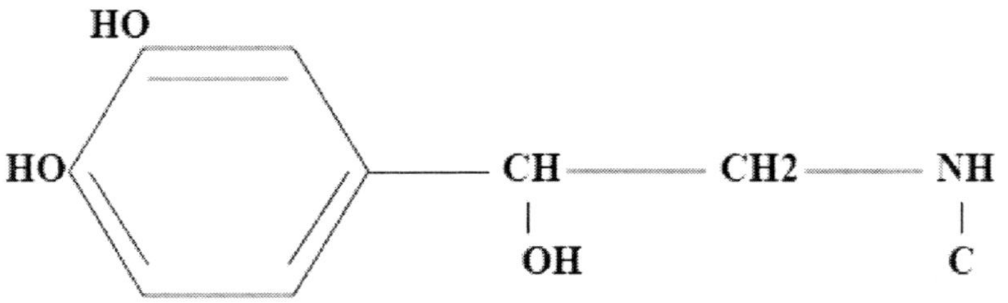

Epinephrine

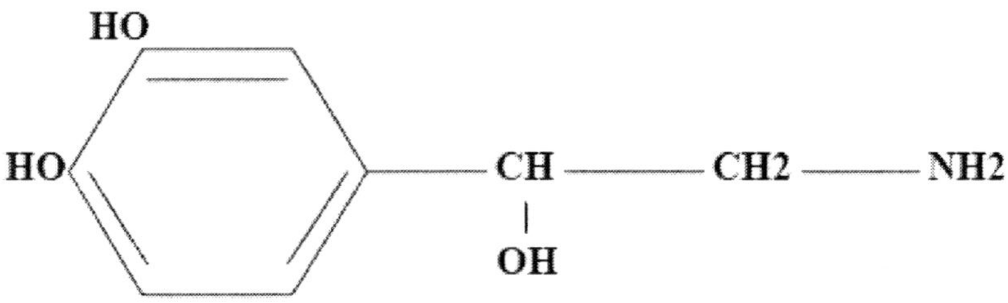

Norepinephrine

Plasma concentrations of epinephrine and norepinephrine usually reflect adrenal medullary secretion and sympathetic nerve activity. Several factors, which are usually related to exercise, mental stress, electrolyte balance, smoking and age [5–6], can stimulate the feed-back mechanism of catecholamine production, metabolism, uptake and excretion.

Physiologically [7–10], catecholamines may have two effects: a direct effect, particularly towards cardiovascular system, and a indirect effect causing changes in hormone secretion and blood flow distribution (Table 5.1.).

Table 5.1. Physiological effects of catecholamines

Direct effect	- Cardiovascular system:
	Vasoconstriction
	Increased heart rate
	Increased myocardial contractility
	Increased conduction velocity
	Enhanced cardiac output
	Venoconstriction
	Increased oxygen consumption
	Hypertension.
Indirect effect	-Endocrine system:
	Renin, insulin,
	glucagone, calcitonin, parathormone,
	thyroxin, gastrin, erythropoietin, sex
	hormone regulation or competition.
	-Blood flow redistribution

Catecholamines influence all the major systems of the body. Their effects, primarily for epinephrine, are very quick if compared with hormone activity of other endocrine glands. Therefore, alterations may seem acute after exposure to a standard or harmful stimulus. Such a property tends to explain the negative effects of the catecholamines on target organs after acute passive smoking exposure that must be considered a strong factor of adrenergic stimulation [11–14]. Moreover, increased levels of catecholamines can be dosed immediately before exercise since the mental stress that precedes exercise performance can induce a raise in these metabolites.

A large variety of hemodynamic and metabolic effects is the response of cardiovascular system to those functional stimuli that cause catecholamine excess. Briefly, the result of the stimulus depends on the type of adrenoreceptor involved. Two types of adrenoreceptors exist, α adrenoreceptors and β adrenoreceptors, the activity of which causes different responses in cardiovascular system.

Catecholamines increase heart rate and myocardial contraction by a β stimulation. On the contrary, vasoconstriction is a result of α stimulation. However, vascular bed of the skeletal muscle undergoes vasodilation through the β adrenoreceptor effect. Norepinephrine induces an increase in both systolic and distolic blood pressure levels as a consequence of an amount in vascular tone, while epinephrine usually raises acutely only systolic blood pressure.

The direct effect of catecholamines causes damage on myocardium [15], primarily by changes in autonomic tone, enhanced lipid mobility, calcium overload, free radical production, increased sarcolemmal permeability (table 5.2.).

Table 5.2. Mechanisms responsible for myocardial damage as a direct catecholamine effect

- Change in autonomic tone
- Enhanced lipid mobility
- Calcium overload
- Free radical production

Moreover, myocardial damage can be the result of a sustained increase in myocardial oxygen demand or decrease in myocardial oxygen availability. The first event occurs as a consequence of catecholamine stimulus, while the second recognizes primarily the effects of environmental tobacco smoke exposure [16], although catecholamines may also have a negative influence potentiating the effects.

Foci of myocardial necrosis with contract bands (see Figure 3.3. of Chapter 3) have been observed as a toxic response to catecholamines. They are probably due to a direct effect of catecholamines on cardiac myocytes via calcium overload, although coronary vasoconstriction accompanied to increased heart rate may play an important role. Moreover, focal myocardial necrosis with contract bands has been described [17] in patients affected by intracranial lesions and elevated cerebrospinal fluid pressure. However, these manifestations are a response to catecholamine cardiotoxicity and are therefore far to appear, following acute or chronic exposure to passive smoking, unless in experimental cardiomyopathy of animals.

ENDOTHELIUM: FUNCTIONAL RESPONSES

Functional effects attributable to vessel bed are primarily identified in changes of endothelial properties, although vascular media and adventitia with vasa vasorum are structures characterized by metabolic events which actively determine the complex physiological response of a vascular tree [18] to stimuli which can induce different manifestations. Among these stimuli, there is undoubtedly passive smoking.

There is evidence that assessing endothelial function can be carried out by both invasive and non-invasive methods. Methods provide details about endothelial capacity to respond to different stimuli as well as the type of response.

Two main methods can be used to assess endothelial function. The first method consists of an endothelium stress test by establishing the endothelial cell response to direct stimulation of the endothelium [19]. It takes advantage of NO release by inducing stimuli and consequent degree of endothelium-dependent vasodilation. The appearance of endothelial dysfunction is a sign of endothelial function impairment with potentially negative progression towards structural lesions. It can be evaluated assessing vascular resistence of forearm vessels following an intra-arterial infusion of an endothelium-dependent vasodilator like acetylcholine [20]. Another non-invasive test using brachial artery ultrasound detection [3, 21] is usually performed to assess endothelium function.

The second method to assess endothelial function measures some peripheral markers which are associated with endothelial dysfunction and the progression of inflammation and atherosclerosis [22]

Table 5.3. summarizes the main methods used to assess endothelial function.

Table 5.3. Main methods used to assess endothelial function

Methods	Principles
1. Endothelial vasomotor testing by coronary Angiography and intracoronary Doppler	Changes in coronary blood flow and coronary vascular resistance.
2. Endothelial vasomotor testing in peripheral vascular bed	Intraarterial infusion of endothelial dependent vasodilators or brachial artery dilation by ultrasonography.
3. Measurement of peripheral markers of endothelial dysfunction	Circulating markers of vascular wall inflammation, NO, endothelin-1.

The assessment of these markers is based on the assumption that their measures permit to establish endothelium reactivity. Indeed, if hemodynamic changes, which tend to increase blood flow, occur in presence of chemical compounds like acetylcholine, normal endothelium produces nitric oxide with consequent vasodilation. On the contrary, when vasoconstrictor stimuli, primarily catecholamines, affect endothelium, its response leads to vasoconstriction. Therefore, an endothelium that maintains its integrity is capable of regulating vasodilator respectively or vasoconstrictor response by a variable secretion of its metabolites.

Moreover, the type of response follows slightly from what can be seen in Figure 5.1. according to the functional characteristics of an applied stimulus.

On the contrary, when a factor, usually mechanical or chemical stimuli, determines an altered response of the endothelial function with decreased vessel dilation and increased contraction, endothelial dysfunction occurs. It may be transient followed by endothelial property restoration to which endothelial progenitor cells seems to contribute actively [23].

Endothelial progenitor cells are primitive cells made in the bone marrow that can enter the bloodstream and then reach those blood vessel areas where an injury has produced damage. Therefore, endothelial progenitor cell function is to help damage repair. Consequently, depletion in their number may contribute to blood vessel disease.

The exact role of these cells in endothelial injury restoration is unclear. In the past, the regeneration of an injured endothelium was attributed to migration and regeneration of endothelial progenitor cells. On the contrary, recent studies [24–28] would demonstrate that additional factors may actively contribute to injured endothelium regeneration. Therefore, circulating endothelial progenitor cells would have a lower importance than that which has been assigned them. Data would indicate that there might be at least two different types of circulating cells that primarily are capable to induce endothelial regeneration, specifically, cells coming from bone marrow as well as non bone marrow cells. The latter cells could arise from either extra bone-marrow sources, namely stem cells living into different tissues, or vessel wall-derived endothelial cells.

Nicotine and the complex of its metabolites would seem to influence both number and activity of circulating endothelial progenitor cells with augmentation and enhanced functional activity of them at relatively low concentrations, while citotoxicity was observed at a higher metabolite concentration [29]. Since nicotine is an active metabolite of the exposure to passive smoking, we can deduce that exposure to environmental tobacco smoke may interfere negatively with the activity of the circulating endothelial progenitor cells, reducing the process of endothelial revascularization and then contributing to maintain endothelial dysfunction.

Endothelial restoration after a damaging stimulus needs a series of complex phenomena to maintain its integrity, the loss of which causes transient or prolonged endothelial dysfunction. As we can see, passive smoking by means of its metabolites, particularly nicotine, is capable of damaging every step of those processes that "help" to maintain endothelium integrity and consequently, induce endothelial dysfunction with progression towards atherosclerotic lesion formation.

Effect of Passive Smoking

The toxic effects of passive smoking, capable of causing functional disorders which can be followed by a structural damage on cardiovascular system even following brief exposure of hours or minutes, are reported to be as large as those from chronic active smoking [30]. Moreover, functional disorders begin as early as initial exposure. However, they are usually transient in the first few times of exposure and respond to the passive smoking as indicated for the response of an isolated stimulus in Figure 5.1: functional restoration of the stimulated structure at the same baseline level after stimulus cessation.

Functional disorders from passive smoking exposure are the result of catecholamine and endothelium stimulation by the main compounds of environmental tobacco. Some of these, particularly nicotine, actively interfere with catecholamine stimulation [1, 31-33], some cause changes in cardiovascular parameters linked to sympathetic or parasympathetic system inducing altered variability in heart rate [34] and hemodynamic changes. Some determine endothelial cell activation by triggering a mechanism of atherosclerosis originally functional but later structural [35]. Moreover, a direct activity of carbon monoxide [33 , 36 – 37], capable to induce a series of changes which recognize either a functional mechanism or later structural changes, should be considered when the functional disorders of cardiovascular system due to passive smoking exposure are analyzed.

It has been well shown that nicotine is the most important factor triggering cardiovascular events initially by a sympathetic discharge [1].

Four main sources (table 5.4.) release catecholamine after nicotine stimulation: sympathetic nerve endings, neurotransmitters within the myocardium, adrenal medulla and chromaffin tissue. The first two structures release primarily norepinephrine, while the latter two mainly epinephrine, but also norepinephrine. By doing so, they respond early to nicotine stimulation but may also prolonge their response in time.

Table 5.4. Structures involved in catecholamine release following nicotine stimulation

Structure	Main Metabolite
Simpathetic nervous endings	Norepinephrine
Intramyocardial neurotransmitters	Norepinephrine
Adrenal medulla	Epinephrine
Chromaffin tissue	Epinephrine, Norepinephrine

The increase in hemodynamic parameters, heart rate and systolic blood pressure are related to plasma nicotine concentrations [31–33]. Moreover, a study of Benowitz and coworkers [38] found that nicotine infusion achieved plasma concentrations of catecholamines and caused increase in heart rate and hemodynamic response similar to those of cigarette smoking up to a limit, beyond which there was no further increase in stimulated parameters. Increased catecholamine concentration, due to nicotine stimulation, was shown by Cryer and coworkers [39], and Hill and Wynder [40].

Experimentally, evidence shows that the release of catecholamines by nicotine is mediated by nicotine receptors [41].

The unsolved question is still the same today-which of the structures listed in Table 5.4. plays a more significant role in inducing prevailingly catecholamine release after nicotine stimulation. Data would suggest an active role of sympathetic neurotransmitters for norepinephrine and adrenal medulla for epinephrine [39].

Acute exposure to passive smoking may reduce heart rate variability [34]. Heart rate variability is measured by analyzing the beat to beat variations in heart rate that can be identified by variations in R –R intervals on the electrocardiogram. Impaired heart rate variability relates the possible triggering of malignant arrhythmias as well as sudden cardiac death [30, 34]. Barnoya and Glantz [30] also affirmed that two hour exposure to passive smoking was associated with a 12% reduction in heart rate variability and this reduction could be associated with an increased risk of ventricular fibrillation or tachycardia. Restoration of baseline heart rate variability could be recorded two hours after exposure. Malignant ventricular arrhythmias with possible reproducibilty of themselves have been shown to characterize acute passive smoking exposure especially for those subjects with a pre-existing myocardial infarction [42–43]. Moreover, these troubles are a close consequence of elevated catecholamine release [44], also prevalent among children with dramatic symptoms that characterized the occurence.

The final result of a functional stimulation due to nicotine is a transiently increased demand in oxygen that otherwise tends to maintain elevated levels of catecholamines. By doing so, reduced oxygen availability prolonges catecholamine activity favoring the occurence of those alterations that open the "door" to atherosclerosis. Moreover, as already aforesaid in a previous chapter, nicotine itself plays a strong role in causing atherosclerosis by the large series of anatomical and metabolic alterations like platelet aggregation, blood coagulation-fibrinolysis cascade activation, lipid metabolism changes and endothelial disruption.

Two main statements must always be kept in mind to understand the relationship between nicotine from passive smoking and catecholamine release. Firstly, the nicotine and its metabolites are certain compounds of passive smoking capable of causing cardiovascular damage. Secondly, in passive smoking, their concentration levels usually can be reached during exposure, causing harmful effects since the appearance of functional disorders by induced-catecholamine stimulation need a low dose of toxic substance. Increased response in heart rate and hemodynamic parameters that do not exceed a maximum level, even if higher nicotine concentration occurs [38], seem to demonstrate the truthfulness of the latter statement.

Carbon monoxide usually follows in two ways: it may activate catecholamine release and then induce functional disorders of cardiovascular system; moreover, it can exert a directly toxic influence. Usually however, the latter influence causes more often anatomical changes than functional disorders.

It could be certainly affirmed, without any need of scientific demonstration, that should the effects of carbon monoxide from passive smoking be those which are attributable to gas poisoning, the harm from passive smoking on exposed individuals would reach the strongest, highest level. Then, similar responses characterize poisoning of carbon monoxide and acute exposure to carbon monoxide from passive smoking, being the same gas that acts in both events. What differs in the inducenent of different responses is the degree of plasma concentration as well as environment concentration of the gas that, during experimentally acute exposure to passive smoking, reaches air concentrations of about 30 to 35 ppm with an exposure time of half an hour [45], and lower but repeated levels for many times during each chronic exposure. These are concentrations of the fastest gas and faster than those observed for acute carbon monoxide poisoning. Therefore, those people who are suspicious with regard to the damage caused by tobacco smoke do not recognize the efficacy of the above statement.

Functional disorders of cardiovascular system, due to carbon monoxide exposure, must be carefully assessed to be set as functional disorders since there are not well defined limits between functional alterations and structural alterations as well as acute exposure and chronic exposure and thus leading to the possibility of an incorrect assessment.

Mechanisms by which carbon monoxide causes functional disorders are not fully known. Moreover, as aforesaid, functional stimulation is often the result of combined direct action of the gas on cardiovascular system and activation of adrenergic system.

Findings in selected population groups would indicate [36] that carbon monoxide could act as a stress factor that potentiates other cardiovascular risk factors to impair cardiovascular symptoms. Moreover, the binding with hemoglobin and other proteins causes hypoxia. Hypoxia can be the factor capable to trigger functional alterations since it activates adrenergic system.

In conclusion, data would show that an indirect relationship mediated by hypoxia links carbon monoxide and adrenergic system. Severe, but often transient, impairment of cardiovascular symptoms when carbon monoxide is associated with other cardiovascular risk factors would mean a manifestation of the reduced availability in oxygen. On the contrary, carbon monoxide leads earlier to those structural alterations of cardiovascular system, already described, as atherosclerotic process acceleration, mitochondrial changes, hemorrhagic foci into areas of myocardial necrosis and experimental cardiomyopathy.

Endothelial cell activation is a very important factor of functional disorders.

As it is known, physiologically endothelial function [46] is the result of a balanced response between vasodilator chemicals as nitric oxide and vasoconstrictors as endothelin. Decreased release of nitric oxide following different types of stimuli and consequently, prevailing of vasoconstrictor response cause endothelial dysfunction; that is, as it is well known, an important marker of early vascular damage that leads to atherosclerosis.

Passive smoking is a strong factor capable to induce endothelial dysfunction even after acute exposure [2 – 3, 21]. Moreover, findings of Celermajer and coworkers [47] compared endothelial function in the arteries of three groups of healthy individuals. The first group included active smokers, the second group lifelong nonsmokers who were exposed to environmental tobacco smoke, and the third group consisted of subjects exposed irregularly to passive smoke. Effective exposure to passive smoking consisted of at least one hour per day anywhere: home, work or both environments.

Endothelial function was assessed by vascular ultrasonography measuring vascular reactivity of brachial artery that is established to be a correct marker of the endothelial function. These findings showed that passive smokers had significantly impaired arterial endothelial function with reduced nitric oxide release.

Impaired availability of nitric oxide, the endothelium-derived relaxing factor, can stimulate platelet aggregation [48–49] that initiates that vascular damage leading to atherosclerosis.

Functional disorders of cardiovascular system following passive smoking exposure have been described as an effect of either isolated catecholamine stimulation or endothelial dysfunction alone. Really, there is evidence that usually functional disorders are the consequence of a complex synergy of these two mechanisms capable to exert their action one by one but, at the same time, potentiating their effects by means of the relationship that links them. In response to epinephrine, the endothelium [30] releases endothelin that causes vasoconstriction; then, vasoconstriction induces endothelial dysfunction that otherwise could be caused directly by some components of passive smoking.. As one can see (Figure 5.3.), functional disorders from passive smoking exposure are the result of at least three different factors which interact among them: adrenergic system stimulation, endothelial dysfunction, and endothelial dysfunction induced by catecholamine release. Passive smoking may act on two main levels: catecholamine release and endothelial dysfunction. The third factor, endothelial dysfunction caused by catecholamine, is the result of physio-pathological synergy that correlate these two factors.

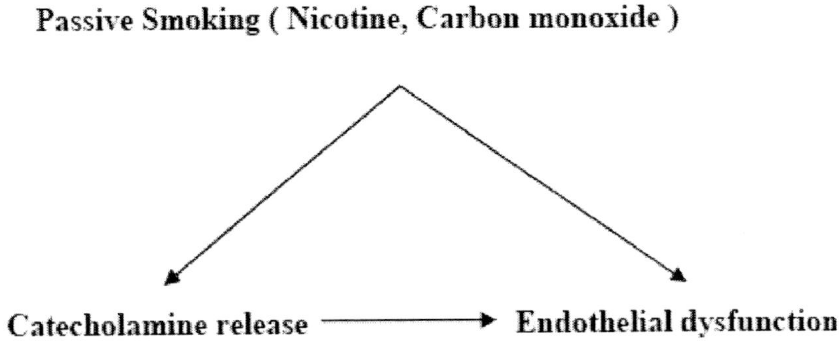

Figure 5.3. Interaction between passive smoking and factors capable to cause functional disorders of cardiovascular system.

Functional changes caused by passive smoking on cardiovascular system tend to improve slightly after a long-term smoking exposure cessation – usually at least one year - especially those manifestations related to endothelial dysfunction. Endothelium-dependent vasodilation has been shown to be better in passive smokers who had ended their exposure when they were compared to current exposed nonsmokers [50], although this parameter was not fully restored in the first group.

Finally, it is noteworthy to confirm again that functional disorders, when they are repeated and left to themselves, lead certainly to the appearance of those anatomical alterations described in chapter 4.

REFERENCES

[1] Ball K, Turner R. Smoking and the heart: The basis for action. *Lancet.* 1974; 2: 822 – 6.

[2] Davis J, Shelton L, Watanabe I, Arnold J. Passive smoking affects endothelium and platelets. *Arch. Intern. Med.* 1989; 149: 386 – 9.

[3] Celermajer DS, Sorensen KE, Gooch VM, Spiegelhalter DJ, Miller OL, Sullivan ID, Lloyd JK, Deanfield JE. Non-invasive detection of endothelial dysfunction in children and adults at risk of atherosclerosis. *Lancet.* 1992; 340: 1111 – 5.

[4] Axelrod J . The metabolism, storage and release of catecholamines. *Recent. Progr. Hormone Research.* 1965; 21: 597 – 622.

[5] Chalmers JP, West MJ. The nervous system in the pathogenesis of hypertension. In: Robertson JIS ed, *Handbook of hypertension, Clinical Aspects of Essential Hypertension.* Elsevier, Amsterdam 1983; Vol 1: 64 – 96.

[6] Calaresu FR, Yardley CP. Medullary basal sympathetic tone. *Ann. Rev. Physiol.* 1988; 50: 511 – 24.

[7] Anton AH, Sayre DF. A study of the factors affecting the aluminum oxide-trihydroxyindole procedure for the analysis of catecholamines. *J. Pharmacol. Exp. Ther.* 1966; 138: 360 – 74.

[8] Hasking GJ, Esler MD, Jennings JL, Dewar E, Lambert J. Norepinephrine spillover to plasma during steady-state supine bicycle exercise. *Circulation.* 1988; 78: 516 – 21.

[9] Riegger AJG, Liebau G. The renin-angiotensin-aldosterone system, antidiuretic hormone and sympathetic nerve activity in an experimental model of congestive heart failure in the dog. *Clin. Sci.* 1982; 62: 465 – 9.

[10] Breuer HW, Skyschally A, Schulz R, Martin C, Wehr M, Heusch G. Heart rate variability and circulating catecholamine concentrations during steady state exercise in healthy volunteers. *Br. Heart J.* 1993; 70: 144 – 9.

[11] Schievelbein H, Richter F. The influence of passive smoking in the cardiovascular system. *Preventive Medicine.* 1984; 13: 626 – 44.

[12] Glantz SA. Air pollution as a cause of heart disease: Time for action. *J. Am. Coll. Cardiol.* 2002; 39: 943 – 5.

[13] Pope CA 3rd, Eatough DJ, Gold DR, Pang Y, Nielsen KR, Nath P, Verrier RL, Kanner RE. Acute exposure to environmental tobacco smoke and heart rate variability. *Environ. Health Perspect.* 2001; 109: 711 – 6.

[14] Cole CR, Lauer MS, Bigger JT. Clinical assessment of the autonomic nervous system. In: Topol EJ ed. *Textbook of Cardiovascular Medicine,* 2nd ed., Lippincot WilliamsandWilkins, Philadelphia, PA, 2002; 1615 – 32.

[15] Lange RA, Hillis DL. Toxins and the Heart. In: Zipes DP, Libby P, Bonow RO, Braunwald E eds. Braunwald's Heart Disease. *A Textbook of Cardiovascular Medicine,* 7th ed, Elsevier – Saunders, Philadelphia, PA, 2005; 1731 – 40.

[16] Leone A. Relationship between cigarette smoking and other coronary risk factors in atherosclerosis: Risk of cardiovascular disease and preventive measures. *Curr. Pharm. Design.* 2003; 9: 2417 – 23.

[17] Samuels MA. Neurally induced cardiac damage: definition of the problem. *Neurol. Clin.* 1993; 11: 273 – 92.

[18] Herrmann J, Lerman LO, Rodriguez-Porcel M, Holmes DR Jr, Richardson DM, Ritman EL, Lerman A. Coronary vasa vasorum neovascularization precedes epicardial endothelial dysfunction in experimental hypercholesterolemia. *Cardiovasc. Res.* 2001; 51: 762 – 6.

[19] Lerman A, Zeiher AM. Endothelial function: cardiac events. *Circulation.* 2005;111: 363 – 8.

[20] Ganz P, Vita JA. Testing endothelial vasomotor function : nitric oxide, a multipotent molecule. *Circulation.* 2003; 108: 2049 – 53.

[21] Giannini D, Leone A, Di Bisceglie D, Nuti M, Strata G, Buttitta F, Masserini L, Balbarini A. The effects of acute passive smoke exposure on endothelium-dependent brachial artery dilation in healthy individuals. *Angiology.* 2006; 57: T1 – T7 (in press).

[22] Verma S, Buchanan MR, Anderson TJ. Endothelial function testing as a biomarker of vascular disease. *Circulation.* 2003; 108: 2054 – 9.

[23] Rafii S, Lyden D. Therapeutic stem and progenitor cell transplantation for organ vascularization and regeneration. *Nat. Med.* 2003; 9: 702 – 12.

[24] Shi Q, Rafii S, Wu MH, Wijelath ES, Yu C, Ishida A, Fujita Y, Kothary S, Mohle R, Sauvage LR, Moore MA, Storb RF, Hammond WP. Evidence for circulating bone marrow-derived endothelial cells. *Blood.* 1998; 92: 362 – 7.

[25] Hillebrands JL, Klatter FA, van Dijk WD, Rozing J. Bone marrow does not contribute substantially to endothelial-cell replacement in transplant atherosclerosis. *Nat. Med.* 2002; 8: 194 – 5.

[26] Walter DK, Rittig K, Bahlmann FH, Kirchmair R, Silver M, Murayama T, Nishimura H, Losordo DW, Asahara T, Isner JM. Statin therapy accelerates reendothelization: a novel effect involving mobilization and incorporation of bone marrow-derived endothelial progenitor cells. *Circulation.* 2002; 105: 3017 – 24.

[27] Werner N, Junk S, Laufs U, Link A, Walenta K, Bohm M, Nickering G. Intravenous transfusion of endothelial progenitor cells reduces neointima formation after vascular injury. *Circ. Res.* 2003; 93: e17 – e24.

[28] Kaushal S, Amiel GE, Guleserian KJ, Shapira OM, Perry T, Sutherland FW, Rabkin E, Moran AM, Schoen FJ, Atala A, Soker S, Bischoff J, Mayer JE Jr. Functional small-diameter neovessels created using endothelial progenitor cells expanded ex vivo. *Nat. Med.* 2001; 7: 1035 – 40.

[29] Wang XX, Zhu JH, Chen JZ, Shang YP. Effects of nicotine on the number and activity of circulating endothelial progenitor cells. *J. Clin. Pharmacol.* 2004; 44: 881 – 9.

[30] Barnoya J, Glantz SA. Cardiovascular effects of secondhand smoke. Nearly as large as smoking. *Circulation.* 2005; 111: 2684 – 98.

[31] Koch A, Hoffmann K, Steck W, Horsch A, Hengen N, Morl H, Harenberg J, Spohr U, Weber E. Acute cardiovascular reactions after cigarette smoking. *Atherosclerosis.* 1980; 35: 67 – 75.

[32] Pachinger O, Hellberg KD, Bing RJ. The effect of nicotine, propranolol, phentolamine and hexamethonium on the coronary microcirculation of the cat. *J. Clin. Pharmacol.* 1972; 12: 432 – 9.

[33] Spohr U, Harenberg J, Walter E, Augustin J, Morl H, Koch A, Weber E. Smoking-induced effects on circulatory and metabolic variables with respect to plasma nicotine and COHb levels. In: Greenhalgh RM ed., *Smoking and Arterial Disease.* Pitman Medical, London 1981; 98 – 106.

[34] Brook RD, Franklin B, Cascio W, Hong Y, Howard G, Lipsett M, Luepker R, Mittleman M, Samet J, Smith SC Jr, Tager I. Air pollution and cardiovascular disease: a statement for healthcare professionals from the Expert Panel on Population and Prevention Science of the American Heart Association. *Circulation.* 2004; 109: 2655 – 71.

[35] Glantz S, Parmley W. Even a little secondhand smoke is dangerous. *JAMA.* 2001; 286: 462 – 3.

[36] Anderson EW, Andelman RJ, Strauch JM, Fortuin NJ, Knelson JK. Effect of low-level carbon monoxide exposure on onset and duration of angina pectoris. *Ann. Intern. Med.* 1973; 79: 46 – 50.

[37] Turino GM. Effect of carbon monoxide on the cardiorespiratory system. Carbon monoxide toxicity: Physiology and biochemistry. *Circulation.* 1981; 63: 253A – 9A.

[38] Benowitz NL, Jacob P III, Jones RT, Rosenberg J. Interindividual variability in the metabolism and cardiovascular effects of nicotine in man. *J. Pharmacol. Exp. Ther.* 1982; 221: 368 – 72.

[39] Cryer PE, Haymond MW, Santiago JV, Shah SD. Norepinephrine and epinephrine release and adrenergic mediation of smoking-associated hemodynamic and metabolic events. *N. Engl. J. Med.* 1976; 295: 573 – 7.

[40] Hill P, Wynder EL. Smoking and cardiovascular disease. Effect of nicotine on the serum epinephrine and corticoids. *Am. Heart J.* 1974; 87: 491 – 6.

[41] Westfall TC, Brasted M. The mechanism of action of nicotine on adrenergic neurons in the perfused guinea-pig heart. *J. Pharmacol. Exp. Ther.* 1972; 182; 409 – 18.

[42] Leone A, Bertanelli F, Mori L, Fabiano P, Bertoncini G. Ventricular arrhythmias by passive smoke in patients with pre-existing myocardial infarction. *J. Am. Coll. Cardiol.* 1992; 19: 256A.

[43] Leone A. Passive smoking causes cardiac alterations in post-MI subjects. *Int. J. Smoking Cessation.* 1996; 3: 42 – 3.

[44] Coumel P, Fidelle J, Lucet V, Attuel P, Bouvrain Y. Catecholamine-induced severe ventricular arrhythmias with Adam-Stokes syndrome in children : Report of four cases. *Br. Heart J.* 1978; 40 (Suppl): 28 – 37.

[45] Leone A, Mori L, Bertanelli F, Fabiano P, Filippelli M. Indoor passive smoking: its effects on cardiac performance. *Int. J. Cardiol.* 1991; 8: 247 – 52.

[46] Cosentino F, Luscher TF. Effects of blood pressare and glucose on endothelial function. *Curr. Hypertens. Rep.* 2001; 3: 79 – 88.

[47] Celermajer DS, Adams MR, Clarkson P, Robinson J, McCredie R, Donald A, Deanfield JE. Passive smoking and impaired endothelium-dependent arterial dilatation in healthy young adults. *N. Engl. J. Med.* 1996; 334: 150 – 4.

[48] Cooke JP, Tsao RS. Is NO an endogenous antiatherogenic molecule? *Arterioscler. Thromb.* 1994; 14: 653 – 5.

[49] Deanfield J. Passive smoking and early arterial damage. *European Heart Journal.* 1996; 17: 645 – 6.

[50] Raitakari OT, Adams MR, McCredie RJ, Griffiths KA, Celermajer DS. Arterial endothelial dysfunction related to passive smoking is potentially reversible in healthy young adults. *Ann. Intern. Med.* 1999; 130:578 – 81.

Chapter 6

METABOLIC DISORDERS

ABSTRACT

There is a strong relationship between passive smoking exposure and some metabolic parameter changes capable to increase the risk of cardiovascular events.

Passive smoking influences negatively coagulation-fibrinolysis cascade at any level, although it acts primarily on those pathways that are most important for an effective clot formation: endothelial metabolites, platelet metabolites, and fibrinogen.

Endothelial dysfunction, caused by prevailing vasoconstrictor metabolites as a response to different environmental tobacco smoke compounds, particularly nicotine, triggers those changes that activate coagulation process, platelet alterations, and fibrinogen. The latter increases its plasma concentrations and together with fibrin framework strengthens clot thickness. Therefore, after exposure to passive smoking, the whole coagulation cascade activates the thrombus formation pathway. The risk of thrombotic cardiovascular events increases its frequency with more severe atherosclerotic alterations if compared to similar events in nonsmokers.

Changes in haemostatic metabolites caused by smoking exposure appear to be related to female sex, especially for those women who use oral contraceptives.

Changes in lipoprotein metabolites have been seen after chronic smoking exposure. Reduced levels of HDL-Cholesterol, a metabolite that prevents atherosclerosis, were shown to be accompanied by an increase of pro-atherogenic LDL-Cholesterol, increase in its oxidation and, therefore, formation of free oxygen radicals that contributed to maintain a high level of oxidative stress. Changes in lifestyle, physical activity and especially, dietary antioxidant supplementation, as well as control of other major cardiovascular risk factors may attenuate stress oxidation.

Glucose intolerance and insulin resistance syndrome would always seem to be newer risk factor for cardiovascular events since they potentiate their effects following passive smoking exposure.

In conclusion, passive smoking induce metabolic changes in coagulation-fibrinolysis cascade, lipid, and glucose parameters that all together lead to atherosclerosis and thrombosis, with consequently a higher rate of cardiovascular events.

Keywords: Passive smoking, Coagulation-fibrinolysis mechanism(s), fibrinogen, Lipid change(s), HDL-Cholesterol, LDL-Cholesterol Glucose intolerance, Insulin resistance syndrome, Free radical(s), Oxidative stress, Antioxidant supplementation.

Metabolic disorders, which maybe caused by exposure to passive smoking, have reflexes on cardiovascular system for what is concerning the different metabolites involved in coagulation-fibrinolysis cascade, lipid metabolism, glucose metabolism with insulin resistance, antioxidant substances. All these metabolites can change their properties under passive smoking stimulation and therefore act as substances capable to induce cardiovascular damage.

Metabolites of Coagulation-Fibrinolysis Cascade

For many years, a relationship between passive smoking and haemostatic metabolites have been well identified [1–7]. Changes in these chemicals have been associated with risk of arterial thrombotic disease, venous thrombotic disease, and ischaemic heart disease [8–13]. When some of them increased, their concentration or function was altered. Severe clinical and pathological manifestations (table 6.1.) related to coagulation-fibrinolysis cascade changes ,can be observed after smoking exposure.

Table 6.1. Main clinical events predisposing to thrombosis related to smoking exposure

1. Platelet disorders
2. Cardiovascular disorders
3. Renal artery diseases
4. Hematologic diseases
5. Immunologic diseases
6. Liver diseases
7. Infective diseases
8. Endocrine diseases
9. Neoplasms with metastatic emboli
10. Spontaneous thrombo-embolic events

Usually, cardiovascular system, which is considered a target organ of the exposure to smoking [4 – 5; 9 – 13; 14 – 23], has involved in hemostatic metabolite changes.

Similar, although quantitatively different, responses characterize smokers, nonsmokers, quitting smokers, men and/ or women who meet cigarette smoking exposure. Complex changes in haemostatic factors may be attributed to the action of many chemical compounds that are usually concentrated and condensed into tobacco mixture [24], mainly nicotine and carbon monoxide, that play a synergy in their action similar to that which occurs with regard to responses of other types after passive smoking exposure.

Studies [25 – 28] identify a large series of changes in chemical metabolites of hemostasis that can cause primarily platelet adhesiveness and aggregation, leukocyte count changes, fibrinogen level increase, plasma viscosity and T-cell function alterations.

A concise description of the main mechanisms of coagulation-fibrinolysis is suitable to be reported for a better understanding the effects of passive smoking exposure on hemostatic metabolites.

MECHANISMS OF COAGULATION-FIBRINOLYSIS

Physiologic mechanisms of coagulation-fibrinolysis [29] derive from the interaction of different factors listed in Table 6.2. Blood vessel, platelet, and plasma factor combined play a basic role for the formation and dissolution of blood clots, the first step of which recognizes, initially, a mechanism of vasoconstriction as a consequence of an injury affecting vascular endothelium. However, the exact mechanism by which blood coagulation is initiated is not well established, and newer chemical components are always found to be involved in the mechanism of coagulation.

Table 6.2. Main steps and their interactions in blood coagulation-fibrinolysis

Steps	Results
1. Vasoconstriction	Reduced blood flow to injured area
2. Thrombin with platelet activation/aggregation	Unstable and transient platelet plug
3. Fibrinogen platelet interaction	Platelet clumping
4. Platelet release of chemical factors adenosine-5-diphosphate, ADP, TXA2, serotonin, phospholipids, lipoproteins	Coagulation-fibrinolysis cascade
5. Fibrinogen to fibrin	Fibrin mesh - white thrombus with only platelets-; red thrombus-with red cells
6. Plasmin	Clot dissolution and lysis

Two pathways lead to the formation of fibrin clot: 1. Intrinsic pathway and 2. Extrinsic pathway. A similar mechanism of vasoconstriction initiates these processes that converge together to clot formation. Then, clot lysis is activated by plasmatic factors usually named fibrinolytic system.

Vascular constriction is the result of a vessel injury caused by stimuli of different type. Then, platelet adhesion, interaction of platelets with a nonplatelet structure such as vascular endothelium, platelet activation and secretion, plasma factor interaction occur.

Chemically, the blood coagulation system is a proteolyitic enzyme cascade [30-33]. Enzymes are present in the plasma as inactive zymogens which on activation undergo lytic cleavage to release active metabolites. The production of thrombin, which can convert soluble fibrinogen into fibrin is the final step of both intrinsic and extrinsic pathways that potentiate their action.

Intrinsic Patway

This phase is activated when blood comes into contact with vessel endothelium and its vascular surface is damaged by injuries of a different type. Quantitatively, this pathway results in the most important phenomenon to initiate coagulation, although it is far from clot formation that occurs quickly in time to stop bleeding.

Different metabolic factors – Hageman factor (factor XII), factor XI, prekallikrein, high molecular weight kininogen – are involved in the pathway activation.

Hageman factor (zymogen) is converted to its active form by a limited proteolysis [34]. When activated, Hageman factor catalyses the conversion of factor XI to factor XIa in presence of two other proteins [35–36]: prekallikrein, converted to kallikrein by activated Hageman factor, and high molecular weight kininogen which optimizes the reaction binding to both prekallikrein and factor XI. Activated factors XIa, XIIa, and kallikrein are serine proteases, like many of the system complement enzymes. The intrinsic pathway could also contribute to the factor X activation, that usually occurs during extrinsic phase. Factor X is the crossroad between intrinsic and extrinsic pathways. It is activated by a group of blood constituents such as activated factor IX, factor VIII, calcium, and phospholipids produced by platelet surface where the phenomenon usually takes place.

Extrinsic Pathway

Clotting cascade may be alternatively activated throughout this way.

This phase provides a second pathway to initiate blood coagulation by converting factor VII to an active protease. Factor III, a tissue factor which is present in most human cells bound to cell membrane, forms a complex with factor VII in presence of calcium. Factor VII and three other coagulation proteins synthesized in the liver – factor II (prothrombin), IX, and X- need calcium and vitamin K for their activity. The activation process for tissue factor is not yet clear. However, once activated factor III together with factor VII and calcium rapidly activate factor X.

Extrinsic pathway provides a rapid response to tissue injury and its main function is to increase the activity of intrinsic pathway. The complex interactions between intrinsic system and extrinsic system, as well as final clot formation, are schematized in Figure 6.1.

The end consequence of both intrinsic and extrinsic pathways is the clot formation by thrombin production for the conversion of fibrinogen to fibrin. This phase is usually followed by clot dissolution and lysis.

A series of biochemical reactions characterizes clot lysis. The fibrinolytic system is essential for removing fibrin deposits in excess and determining vessel lumen patency.

The main metabolite of fibrinolytic system is plasminogen present in human plasma. Conversion of plasminogen to plasmin is a consequence of a number of chemical agents commonly called plasminogen activators. The main plasminogen activator in humans is a 70-kDa serine proteinase formed by a single polypeptide chain. This factor is known as tissue-type plasminogen activator (t-PA). t-PA is converted by plasmin to a two- chain form by hydrolytic mechanisms. Other different plasminogen activators, such as single-chain urokinase-type plasminogen activator, play a significant role in regulating fibrinolytic system. Fibrin clot lysis is a result of interaction between concentrations of fibrin in the clot, natural plasminogen activators, and endogenous plasminogen inhibitors activity in balance, physiologically among themselves (Figure 6.2.).

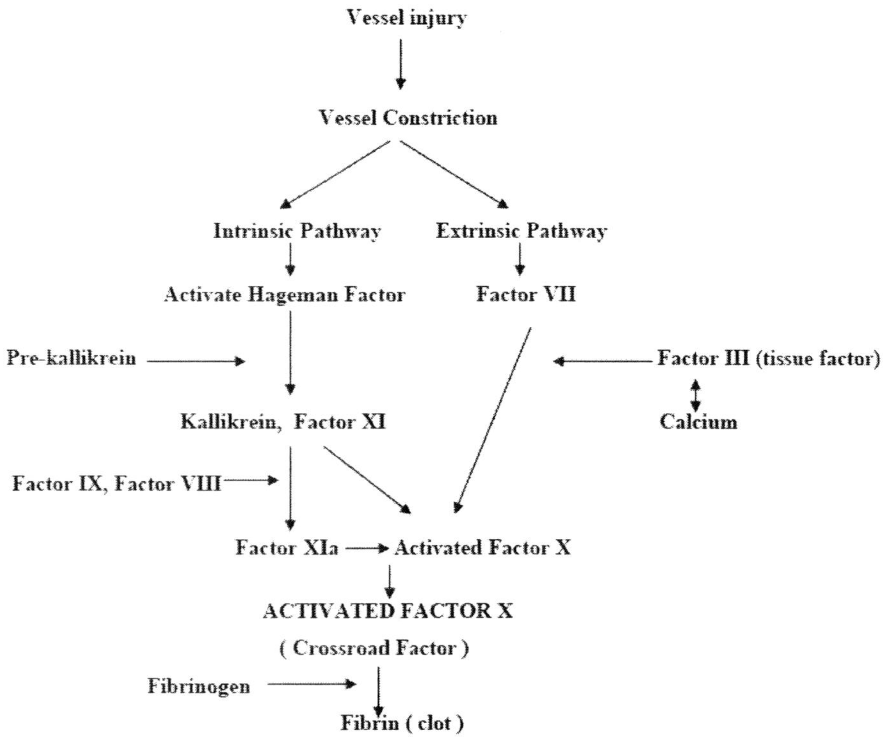

Figure 6.1. Schematic description of the complex phenomena involving the main hemostatic metabolites in coagulation-fibrinolysis cascade.

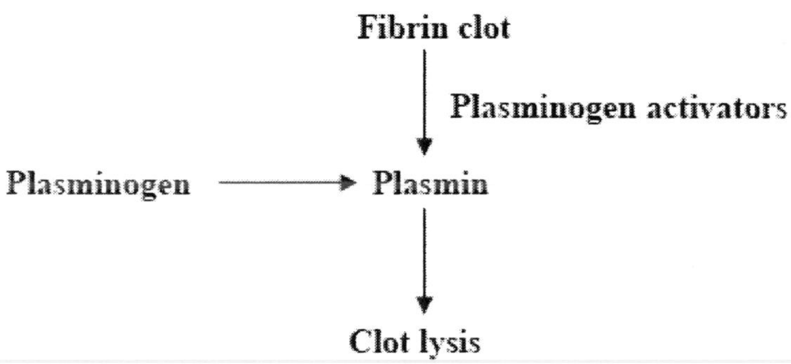

Figure 6.2. Schematic description of clot lysis.

The whole coagulation-fibrinolysis cascade is regulated, physiologically, to avoid the hemorrhages and maintain vessel lumen patency that is a basic component to warrant blood rheology. Therefore, a loss of the balance between these two functions, that passive smoking exposure can chronically induce, triggers those metabolic changes in any step of coagulation-fibrinolysis system with possible appearance particularly of thrombotic manifestations that negatively affect the cardiovascular system [37 – 41].

EFFECTS OF COAGULATION-FIBRINOLYSIS METABOLITE CHANGES DUE TO SMOKING EXPOSURE

A complex relationship exists between cigarette smoking, haemostatic metabolites and cardiovascular system. Smoking exposure may damage cardiovascular system, whether directly or by inducing changes in haemostatic metabolites, which are strong risk factors for heart and blood vessels and may lead to thrombosis. Undoubtedly, severe thrombotic alterations affect coronary arteries of smokers compared to nonsmokers [10, 20, 42]. In their turn, never smokers exposed to environmental tobacco smoke show vascular pathology of a more severe degree than that experienced by non-exposed never smokers. Thrombosis is always a consequence of the interaction of the three components [43-44] of the Virchov triad (see chapter 3): altered vessel wall, impaired blood flow, and changes in haemostatic metabolite function. Moreover, atherothrombotic complications mainly affect the coronary arteries, cerebrovascular arteries, and arteries of systemic circulation [45] which are sites negatively influenced by passive smoking.

Understanding how and where passive smoking impairs haemostatic metabolites and then potentiates its harmful effect on cardiovascular system through this way is easy if the main steps of coagulation-fibrinolysis cascade are analyzed. As indicated above, endothelium changes, platelet adhesiveness and aggregation, fibrinogen activation are the most important phases that lead to clot formation. Each factor capable of influencing these parameters causes changes in clot characteristics. Both active smoking and passive smoking impair endothelial function [13, 21, 39, 46], exacerbate platelet adhesiveness and aggregation [21, 47 – 51], increase plasma fibrinogen levels [2, 7, 21, 52].

Normal endothelium is a structure that is not reactive with the constituents of circulating blood. On the contrary, altered endothelium and denudated vascular surfaces, especially those covered by prosthetic material, activate those pathways which lead to thrombi formation.

Endothelial dysfunction is the result of a complex interaction of factors [53] causing endothelium activation, which involves blunted endothelium-dependent vasodilation-vasodilator change as well as inflammatory processes [45, 54 – 55] extending to the milieu within the whole vasculature. Experimental studies conducted in humans [48, 56] showed that exposure to both types of tobacco smoke, active smoking and secondhand smoking, increased the appearance of anuclear endothelial cells in the blood. These structures are the result of endothelial damage, which can be considered the initiating step of atherosclerosis.

After the disruption of endothelial layer by an injury factor – mechanical, chemical or inflammatory - blood coagulation initiates by platelet activation, and interaction of activated platelets, vessel wall and plasma metabolites.

There is evidence [21, 50] in one experiment that nonsmokers and smokers were asked to smoke two cigarettes. Smoker platelets, at the beginning of smoking, were maximally activated and did not show further activation at the end of smoking. On the contrary, nonsmoker platelets increased their activation as a response to cigarette smoke. Moreover, measured platelet activity [50] in both smokers and nonsmokers before and after they sat in a room for 20 minutes where cigarettes had been smoked just before the experiment started, showed no significant change in smoker platelets, whereas nonsmoker platelets had a significantly major activity. Therefore, these experiments would provide a strong evidence that smoking, yet passive smoke, can impair coagulation-fibrinolysis cascade by platelet activation, the second step (Table 6.2.) in clot formation and then activate those hemostatic metabolites that continue the process.

Biochemically, studies of cigarette- smoke extract on the effects of platelet activity suggest that cigarette smoking compounds increase platelet-activating factor by influencing the activity of the plasma enzyme platelet-activating factor acetylhydrolase [57], which reduces platelet activity by neutralizing platelet-activating factor. After adhesion of the platelets, they become deformed and then aggregate more intensively exposing surface-platelet factors that interact with plasma factors to bind and activate fibrinogen.

Studies [55, 58] emphasize that tissue factor is a prominent component of plaque lesions. Unstable plaques have intensive tissue factor activity. Tissue factor, as mentioned above, is the crossroad of coagulation-fibrinolysis cascade (Figure 6.1.) leading to formation of thrombin and fibrin.

The effects of fibrinogen-fibrin and its split products in the vessel wall, although widely studied, need further findings.

There are different clinical studies which underline that increased concentration of intravascular fibrin is an indicator of severity of atherosclerosis in peripheral artery diseases [9, 45, 59 – 64]. Moreover, all these studies would seem to show that the components of tobacco smoke, especially nicotine and carbon monoxide, affect mainly endothelium, platelets, and coagulation-fibrinolysis cascade.

Carbon monoxide [65] is a gas that is quickly absorbed into the blood, reducing blood capacity to carry oxygen. Carbon monoxide either clinically or experimentally, affects different components of the blood, tissues, and organs [10-11, 15, 19, 66 – 71].

Nicotine and its metabolites harm the heart and blood vessels by biochemical and anatomical changes [39]. Some of these changes are related to atherogenic and thrombogenic risk such as increased cholesterol levels, low-density lipoproteins, triglycerides, total white, red, and platelet blood cell count, hematocrit, prothrombin time, partial thromboplastin time and fibrinogen. Table 6.3. shows the negative effects of the two chemicals on metabolic parameters. As one can see, chemical substances related to different metabolic chains are influenced by the main components of passive smoking.

Table 6.3. Negative metabolic effects of nicotine and carbon monoxide

Nicotine	Carbon monoxide
Increased prothrombin time	Increased carboxyhemoglobin
Increased thromboplastin time	
Increased fibrinogen levels	
Increased total Cholesterol	
Increased LDL-Cholesterol	
Increased Triglycerides	
Decreased HDL-Cholesterol	

These metabolic changes, particularly of the haemostatic metabolites, occur to different levels: vascular level , endothelial level, cellular level, and plasmatic level. Establishing the exact role and interaction among these levels is yet unclair. From time to time, there is a major involvement of endothelium and platelets particularly in the presence of association between smoking exposure and hypertension, major involvement of lipid metabolism and fibrinogen if an association between smoking exposure and lipid profile alterations with fatty plaque formation exists, and, once more, major involvement of plasma metabolites when a direct toxicity of chemical compounds of smoking affects cardiovascular system.

A chemical that is not a metabolite, in the true sense of the word, but permits a physiological response of several metabolic compounds, is calcium.

Calcium deposits have been found into the arterial wall together with a major incidence and extension of thrombi [72–83]. These observations are a close effect of haemostatic parameter alterations and affect cardiovascular system of active smokers and exposed never smokers with a significantly major incidence, when these two groups are compared with non-exposed never smokers. Moreover, these anatomical changes usually have an unfavorable prognosis for affected subjects.

Leone et al. [73] conducted an histopathologic study on the myocardium and coronary vessels of subjects who died from acute myocardial infarction and did not have any other coronary risk factors, unless cigarette smoking. Structural alterations observed in these individuals were compared with similar alterations of nonsmokers who were used as a control group. Then, heavier and markedly more extensive lesions characterized the smokers, and these lesions related well to haemostatic system impairment with a primary involvement of platelets and endothelium. Some effects could be attributed to hemostatic metabolite changes caused by passive smoking exposure, although at a lower level.

Auerbach et al. [20] found more advanced narrowings of coronary arteries in smokers, particularly heavy smokers when compared to nonsmokers. Smoking promoted the formation of fatty plaques on the surface of blood vessels and thickening of the small coronary vessels.

Smokers who survived a first acute myocardial infarction showed a cardiovascular damage due to smoking components with a prevalence of atherosclerotic alterations of heart and coronary vessels in the studies of Pohjola et al. [84], Wilhelmsson et al. [19], Daly et al., Jenkins et al., and Vliestra et al. [85–87]. These alterations could be pathogenetically influenced by hemostatic metabolite changes that usually act as thrombogenic factors.

Therefore, smoking exposure is undoubtedly strongly associated with an increased incidence of atherosclerotic events, the large majority of which can be conducted to previous coagulation-fibrinolysis cascade alterations which interact actively with other similar thrombogenic changes caused by those functional and biochemical substances already analyzed that worsen cardiovascular system responses.

Passive Smoking, Hemostatic Metabolite Changes and Women

Attention needs to be given to the relationship between smoking exposure, haemostatic metabolite alterations and female gender. Really, the endocrine constellation of women must be known to understand the different effects of women and men to smoking exposure. The risk for cardiovascular events in some age is heavier in women than that in men. This condition will be further explained in the chapter which will treat the responses to passive smoking exposure of special categories. Table 6.4. lists the main different responses to smoking exposure and haemostatic factors of two sexes.

Table 6.4. Different responses to hemostatic metabolites after smoking exposure in men and women

Men	- Impairment of cardiovascular system with thrombi formation (acute exposure and chronic exposure to smoke)
	- Coagulatin-fibrinolysis cascade impairment with increased fibrinogen (acute exposure and chronic exposure to smoke)
Women	- Impairment of cardiovascular system in older age (acute exposure and chronic exposure to smoke)
	- Coagulation-fibrinolysis cascade impairment with early thrombosis (acute exposure and chronic exposure to smoke and concomitantly oral contraceptive drug use before menopause)
	- Hypertension

Physiologically, sexual hormone constellation protects women from cardiovascular attacks in pre-menopausal state, unless in a limited number of events [88–91]. On the contrary, post-menopausal woman increases of two-three-fold cardiovascular risk when compared with pre-menopausal state.

Oral contraceptives drugs containing a mixture of estrogens and progestogens, that produces a hormonal constellation similar to that found during the luteal phase of an ovulatory menstrual cycle, have to be considered a strong risk for heart and coagulation-fibrinolysis system when they are associated with smoking exposure. That makes men and women different with regard to cardiovascular risk.

The most serious complication of using oral contraceptives is an increased incidence of thromboembolic phenomena at both vascular levels: arteries and veins. Originally, the damage caused by contraceptive drugs, believed to be due to estrogen components, but now there is evidence [92] of a damage due to progestogens.

Cerebrovascular thrombosis and haemorrhage increase their incidence nine-fold and two-fold respectively among women using oral contraceptives, whereas spontaneous incidence of these cerebrovascular events is markedly lower in control groups who did not use the drugs. Smoking exposure furtherly increases the incidence. Same results for thrombophlebitis, pulmonary embolism, and hepatic vein thrombosis characterized passive smoking exposure. Hypertension relates well to use of oral contraceptives raising its incidence to five-fold after a follow-up period of about five years.

Also coronary artery disease is closely related to contraceptive drugs. Angina pectoris and myocardial infarction, more than sudden cardiac death, are seen to affect woman who are habitual smokers.

Estrogens increase serum lipid levels and these alteration are potentiate heavily by associated diabetes mellitus, obesity, and smoking exposure especially in older women. Hemostatic metabolite changes, particularly plasma fibrinogen concentrations, derived from passive smoking exposure contribute actively.

However, one report [93] underlines that use of noncontraceptive estrogens was not associated with an excess risk of acute myocardial infarction. Furthermore, menopausal estrogen therapy has been associated with a protective effect from coronary heart disease death.

On the contrary, users of contraceptive estrogen who smoke or are passively exposed to smoke need a close control being at a greater risk of thromboembolic events [92–95], compared with those users who are not related to smoking exposure.

There are different opinions [96-108] on the relationship between smoking exposure, estrogen use, hormone replacement therapy, and haemostatic metabolites. Some of these studies emphasize an increased risk for cardiac and cerebrovascular events, whereas others confirm that estrogens protect brain and heart from thromboembolic lesions and changes in hemostatic metabolites.

Kurth and coworkers [96] demonstrated in a prospective study that the risk of total haemorrhagic stroke increased in those women who were current cigarette smokers. On the contrary, Hurn and coworkers [97] showed that estrogens could protect the brain from experimental stroke, reducing brain ischaemia and subaracnoidal hemorrhage. However, there is much confusion in an overall analysis of these results, with some papers conducted on heart alone, some on heart and blood vessels, some on brain alone, and finally, some on heart and brain together. Moreover, there is an unclear attribution of the negative effects to active smoking or passive smoking since these two factors are considered as having almost similar activity in different papers and changes in hemostatic metabolites caused by passive smoking exposure were not well divided between pre-menopausal and post-menopausal women.

In my opinion, observations derived from a large series of personal findings on the relationship between active and passive smoking, hemostatic metabolite changes and women exposed suggest a high precaution in using contraceptive drugs only for those pre-menopausal women who are current smokers, especially if heavy smokers, suffering from ischemic cardiovascular disease manifestations.

Lipid Metabolism Changes

In addition to hemostatic metabolite changes, passive smoking exposure is strongly associated with lowering in HDL- Cholesterol that is known to prevent atherosclerosis development [109]. Such an activity is in contrast to what characterizes same classes of chemical compounds where all belongings usually exert a synergistic action. Really, the large majority of lipoproteins has pro-atherosclerotic effects (see also chapter 4).

Physiologically, lipoproteins [110] arise from an interaction between adipose tissue and diet to form fatty acids. Then, these compounds are esterified to tryglicerides into the liver. Some of the fatty acids may be synthesized directly in the liver from acetate. Then, a series of chemical reactions regulated by enzymatic activity determine Cholesterol-lipoprotein formation (Figure 6.3.).

The major lipoproteins are usually classified (Table 6.5.) according to their increasing size and decreasing density in: high-density lipoprotein (HDL), low-density lipoprotein (LDL), very low-density lipoprotein (VLDL), and chylomicron. Intermediate-density lipoproteins (IDL) are often considered in lipoprotetein classification and are placed between LDL and VLDL lipoproteins.

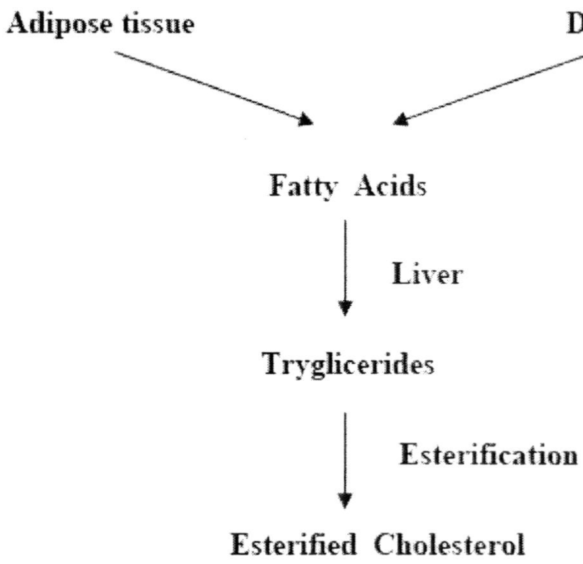

Figure 6.3. Main steps to synthesize Cholesterol in the liver.

Table 6.5. Classes of lipoproteins according to their molecular size and density

Class	Major Lipid Component
Chylomicron	Trygliceride
Very low-density lipoprotein (VLDL)	Trygliceride
Intermediate-density lipoprotein (IDL)	Cholesteryl ester
Low-density lipoprotein (LDL)	Cholesteryl ester
High-density lipoprotein (HDL)	Cholesteryl ester
	Phospholipid

The difference in size, density, and, particularly, in fatty compounds, regulates pro-atherogenic or preventive effects on atherosclerosis development of these molecules.

Passive smoking leads to lower level of HDL-Cholesterol [111-112]. Exposed nonsmokers, particularly women in workplace and home, had HDL-Cholesterol levels higher than those of non exposed never smokers with sometimes similar values of active smokers in different studies [112, 113–114]. Both acute exposure to passive smoking and chronic exposure reach the same effects.

About what is concerning the mechanism by which passive smoking reduces plasma HDL-Cholesterol, there is evidence that LDL- Cholestelol would play an important role [115] (Table 6.6.).

Table 6.6. Main effects of HDL and LDL-Cholesterol on atherosclerotic process

HDL - Cholesterol	LDL - Cholesterol
Inhibition in foam cell formation	Monocyte endothelial cell binding
Prevention LDL Cholesterol oxidation	Foam cell formation
Removing Cholesterol excess (bile)	Oxidant substance production
Inhibition intraendothelial monocyte migration	Fibrous cap formation (atheroma)
Antioxidant property	Endothelial dysfunction
Endothelial function protection	

Oxidized LDL Cholesterol is the major precursor of atherogenesis. Oxidation leads monocytes to bind endothelial cells with consequent migration into the intima of the arterial vessels. As already described (see also Chapter 4), this process leads to foam cell and through different steps, atheroma formation. HDL- Cholesterol develops its preventing effect on atherosclerosis through an inhibition in foam cell formation and prevention of the oxidation to LDL-Cholesterol, as well as preventing endothelial dysfunction. Two main mechanisms act [115–116]. Firstly, HDL-Cholesterol contributes to remove cholesterol excess from blood vessels, moves it into the liver, where cholesterol can be excreted by bile. This process is known as "reverse cholesterol transport". Secondly, HDL-Cholesterol impedes LDL- Cholesterol oxidation, inhibits monocytes migration through endothelial wall, has antioxidant properties. On the contrary, passive smoking not only impedes a regular development of HDL-Cholesterol activity by favoring LDL-Cholesterol oxidation, but also reduces actively plasma HDL-Cholesterol levels. Moreover, acute exposure to passive smoke results in deterioration of serum antioxidant defense [21].

HDL-Cholesterol lowering after exposure to passive smoking has been well identified also in children [117–119]. Moreover, data would suggest that white males who had been exposed to passive smoking could undergo lower HDL-Cholesterol levels than black people or women [119]. However, these data are in contrast with other reports [22, 96 – 98] and therefore, need further findings.

Glucose Metabolism and Insulin Resistance

Smoking may be an independent, modifiable risk factor for non-insulin dependent diabetes mellitus [120]. Findings on both active smokers and passive smokers identified more that passive smoking was associated with an increased risk of developing glucose intolerance [121–124]. Findings [125] found that subjects undergone passive smoking exposure had an intermediate risk to develop glucose intolerance between active smokers and never smokers. This risk was similar to that of previous smokers who stopped smoking. Moreover, racial and sex prevailing was found in exposed never smokers with a major incidence in white people and men.

In conclusion, there is evidence that exposure to passive smoke must be identified as a newer risk factor for glucose intolerance in exposed never smokers, although expanding findings would seem to need a support to this statement.

An indirect stimulation to induce glucose intolerance may be hypothesized by adrenergic effects that link passive smoking and catecholamine release as well as catecholamine release and glucose. Really, passive smoking increases catecholamine release which, in its turn, causes increased glucose levels.

Increased insulin resistance is now recognized as a risk factor for heart disease [126].

Insulin resistance syndrome [127], better named metabolic syndrome (there are, however, some different terms to define this syndrome: syndrome X, dysmetabolic syndrome X, Reaven syndrome), consists of a large series of metabolic disorders characterized by obesity, high blood pressure, changes in lipid profile with elevated LDL-Cholesterol and low HDL-Cholesterol, increased trygliceride concentration, and particularly, high blood insulin levels. The fundamental defect in this syndrome recognizes a different, but elevated, degree of insulin resistance to two levels: adipose tissue and muscle. Insulin resistance syndrome is usually also associated with endothelial dysfunction and changes in those hemostatic metabolites having a prothrombotic effects. Table 6.7. summarizes the main metabolic and clinical characteristics of insulin resistance syndrome.

Table 6.7. Metabolic and clinical characteristics of insulin resistance syndrome

Metabolic characteristics	Clinical manifestations
Hypergliycemia	Type 2 Diabetes mellitus
Hyperinsulinemia	Obesity (mainly abdominal)
Insulin resistance	Chronic sub-clinical inflammation
LDL Cholesterol increase	Ischemic heart disease
Trygliceride increase	Thrombo-embolic disease
HDL-Cholesterol decrease	Endothelial dysfunction
Fibrinogen increase	Atherosclerosis
Other hemostatic metabolite increase	

Epidemiological studies [126, 128] showed that exposure to passive smoking could increase insulin resistance, particularly in women, although this statement was not confirmed by another study [129].

However, the mechanism by which passive smoking can cause a major incidence of ischemic heart disease might be recognized in an increase in insulin resistance that, therefore, is added to other different risk factors to damage cardiovascular system.

Oxidative Metabolic Stress and Antioxidant Supplementation

Oxidative stress is a term used to describe the level of structural damages caused by free oxygen radicals in a cell, tissue or organ. Free oxygen radicals are a group of molecules that derive from oxygen metabolism and exist in all aerobic organisms. Usually, endogenous sources may originate these compounds. Among exogenous sources, smoking exposure in both its forms, active and passive smoking, plays a significant role, but not the strongest, in inducing free oxygen radical formation [130]. Formation is the result of oxidative reactions that characterize intracellular respiratory metabolism [131].

Free oxygen radicals increase their amount after passive smoking exposure [21] and cause natural antioxidant depletion.

All groups of populations negatively feel the action of these compounds associated with antioxidant depletion, being the latter factor that impedes an excessive LDL-Cholesterol oxidation. Children exposed to passive smoking [132] are exposed to oxidative stress at different levels, including atherosclerosis.

The level of oxidative stress is the result of the balance between the rate at which metabolism is damaged and the rate at which it is effectively repaired and then removed (Figure 6.4.).

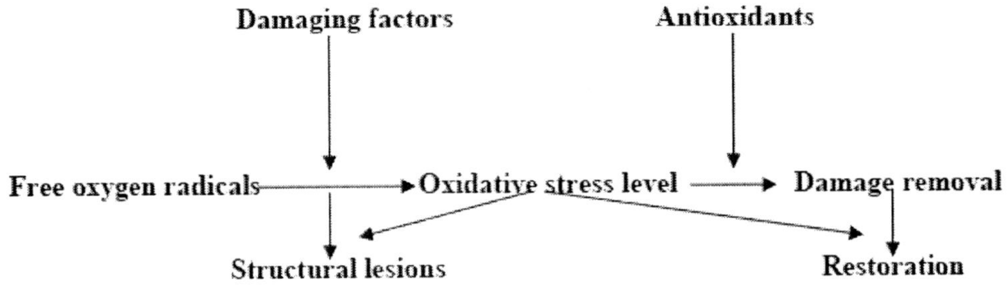

Figure 6.4. Response of oxidative stress to damaging factors and antioxidants.

Antioxidant level is therefore an important mechanism to regulate the damage from oxidative stress following exposure to passive smoking. Both natural antioxidants and antioxidants from dietary supplementation can provide an effective aid to try reducing metabolic damage. However, most often these measures do not reach important results. A "cocktail" of preventive measures could have better effects to control the negative effects of oxidative stress.

Preventive measures against oxidative stress from passive smoking must face at least 3 changes: lifestyle changes consisting particularly, of avoiding smoking exposure and more physical activity, diet supplementation, and control of other major cardiovascular risk factors also using, if it is necessary, drug administration.

Avoiding smoking exposure would be the better way to change the oxidative stress level and then prevent metabolic damage derived from environmental tobacco smoke.

Physical activity, performed regularly, without any excess that could impair oxidative stress, is an effective measure in reducing the degree of damage. Moderate exercise reduces atherosclerosis progression, causes arterial vessel dilatation, determines fall in body weight and probably increases HDL-Cholesterol levels. However, the role of physical activity are not completely clarified, although physical fitness and leisure-time physical activity seem to be associated [133], with encouraging results in preventing cardiovascular damage.

Diet supplementation always recognizes more effective results [134–138].

The composition of the diet has different effects on individuals metabolism with regard to their components. The purpose of dietary measures is to provide those antioxidant substances that can reduce oxidative stress and by doing so,reduce the risk of cardiovascular events.

Different dietary measures have been suggested to control the major manifestations of oxidative stress. Epidemiologic studies have shown that vitamins C and E [134] were found significantly lower in smokers compared to nonsmokers. Moreover, endothelium-dependent vasodilation in chronic smokers could be improved by acute intraarterial administration of vitamin C [135]. In the Health Professionals' follow-up study [136], male subjects taking daily 100 to 250 IU vitamin E supplementation reduced the risk of cardiovascular events. Different results however reached another randomized trial [137]. Finally, in a little group of subjects [138], oral supplementation of vitamin E could attenuate transient impairment of endothelial function after heavy smoking exposure as a consequence of this improvement of the oxidative status, but not chronic endothelial dysfunction. Therefore, one can conclude that among different antioxidants, particularly vitamin C and E, the effects of oxidative stress can be reduced.

The control of other major cardiovascular risk factors, obtained also by pharmacological therapy, could impede the negative effects of oxidative stress primarily when serum LDL-Cholesterol, hypertension, diabetes mellitus and obesity are stably reduced.

References

[1] Kannel WB, Schatzkin A. Risk factor analysis. *Progr. Cardiov. Dis.* 1983; 26: 309 – 332.

[2] Kannel WB, Wolf PA, Castelli WP, D'Agostino RB. Fibrinogen and risk of cardiovascular disease: The Framingham Study. *JAMA.* 1987; 258: 1183 – 6.

[3] Ridker PM, Hennekens CH. Haemostatic risk factors for coronary heart disease. *Circulation.* 1991; 83: 1098 – 1100.

[4] Fowkes FGR. Aetiology of peripheral atherosclerosis. Smoking seems especially important. *BMJ.* 1989; 298: 405 – 6.

[5] Trap-Jensen J. Effects of smoking on the heart and peripheral circulation. *Am. Heart J.* 1988; 115: 263 – 6.

[6] Folts JD, Bonebrake FC. The effects of cigarette smoke and nicotine on platelet thrombus formation in stenosed dog coronary arteries; inhibition with phentolamine. *Circulation.* 1982; 65: 465 – 9.

[7] Meade T, Imeson J, Sterling Y. Effects of changes in smoking and other characteristics in clotting factors and the risk of ischaemic heart disease. *Lancet.* 1987; ii: 986 – 8.

[8] FitzGerald GA, Smith B, Pederson AK, Brash AR. Increased prostacyclin biosynthesis in patients with severe atherosclerosis and platelet activation. *N. Engl. J. Med.* 1984; 310: 1065 – 8.

[9] Lassila R, Laustiola KE. Cigarette smoking and peripheral arterial occlusive disease-evidence for adrenergic connections. *J. Smoking-Related Dis.* 1992; 3: 217 – 23.

[10] Leone A. Cardiovascular damage from smoking: a fact or belief? *Int. J. Cardiol.* 1993; 38: 113 – 7.

[11] Leone A. Cigarette smoking and health of the heart. *J. Roy. Soc. Health.* 1995; 1115: 354 – 5.

[12] Reid DD, Hamilton PJS, McCartney P, Rose G. Smoking and other risk factors in coronary heart disease in British civil servants. *Lancet.* 1976; ii: 979 – 84.

[13] Leone A. Relationship between cigarette smoking and other coronary risk factors in atherosclerosis: risk of cardiovascular disease and preventive measures. *Curr. Pharm. Design.* 2003; 9(29): 2417 – 23.

[14] Sherman CB. Health effects of cigarette smoking. *Clin. Chest. Med.* 1991 Dec; 12(4): 643 – 58.

[15] Leone A. The heart: a target organ for cigarette smoking. *J. Smoking-Related Dis.* 1992; 3: 197 – 201.

[16] Hammond EC, Garfinkel L. Coronary heart disease, stroke, and aortic aneurysm. *Arch. Environ. Health.* 1969; 19: 167 – 82.

[17] Aronow WS. Effect of passive smoking on angina pectoris. *N. Engl. J. Med.* 1978; 299: 21 – 4.

[18] Leone A, Bertanelli F, Mori L, Fabiano P, Bertoncini G. Ventricular arrhythmias by passive smoking in patients with pre-existing myocardial infarction. *J. Am. Coll. Cardiol.* 1992; 3: 256 A.

[19] Wilhelmsson C, Vedin JA, Elmfeldt D, Tibblin G, Wilhelmsen L. Smoking and myocardial infarction. *Lancet.* 1975; 1: 415 – 20.

[20] Auerbach O, Carter HW, Garfinkel L, Hammond EC. Cigarette smoking and coronary heart disease, a macroscopic and microscopic study. *Chest.* 1976; 70: 697 – 705.

[21] Glantz SA, Parmley WW. Passive smoking and heart disease. *JAMA.* 1995; 273 – 1047 – 53.

[22] Wells AJ. Passive smoking as a cause of heart disease. *J. Am. Coll. Cardiol.* 1994; 24: 546 – 54.

[23] Leone A, Giannini D, Bellotto C, Balbarini A. Passive Smoking and Coronary heart disease. *Current Vascular Pharmacology.* 2004; 2: 175 – 82.

[24] Byrd JC. Environmental tobacco smoke. *Medical and legal issues.* Medical Clinics of North America. 1992; 76: 377 – 97.

[25] Imaizumi T, Satoh K, Yoshida H, Kawamura Y, Hiramoto M, Takamatsu S. Effect of cigarette smoking on the levels of platelet-activating factor-like lipid(s) in plasma lipoproteins. *Atherosclerosis.* 1991; 87: 47 – 55.

[26] Becker C, Dubin T. Activation of factor XII glicoprotein by tobacco. *J. Exp. Med.* 1977; 146: 457 – 67.

[27] Saba S, Mason R. Some effects of nicotine on platelets. Thromb Res 1975; 7: 819 – 24.

[28] FitzGerald GA, Oates JA, Novak J. Cigarette smoking and hemostatic function. *Am. Heart J.* 1988; 115: 267 – 71.

[29] Handin RI. Physiology of coagulation: the platelet. In Hematology of Infancy and Childhood, 3d ed., Nathan DG and Oski FA eds; *Philadelphia Saunders.* 1987; 1271 – 92.

[30] Schmidt A. Pflugers Archives 1872; 6: 445 (Quoted by Howell 1935).

[31] Howell WH. Theories of blood coagulation. *Physiology Reviews.* 1935; 15: 435 – 70.

[32] Mcfarlane RG. An enzyme cascade in the blood clotting mechanism and its function as a biochemical amplifier. *Nature.* 1964; 202: 498 – 9.

[33] Davie EW, Ratnoff ED. Waterfall sequence for intensive blood clotting. *Science.* 1964; 145: 1310 – 2.

[34] Rewak SD, Cochrane CG, Bouma BN, Griffin JH. Surface and fluid phase activities of two forms of activated Hageman factor produced during contact activation of plasma. *J. Exp. Med.* 1978; 147: 719 - 29.

[35] Hathaway WE, Belhanson LP, Hathaway HS. Evidence for a new thrombo-plastin factor. Case report, coagulation studies and physicochemical studies. *Blood.* 1965; 26: 521 – 32.

[36] Wuepper KD. Biochemistry and biology of components of the plasma kinin-forming system. In Inflammation: *Mechanisms and Control,* Lepow IH and Ward PA eds; Academic, New York 1972; 93 -117 .

[37] Peto R, Lopez AD, Boreham J, Thun M, Heath C. Mortality from smoking in developed countries: 1950 – 2000. Oxford: Oxford University Press 1994.

[38] Wald NJ, Hackshaw AK. Cigarette smoking: an epidemiological overview. *British Medical Bulletin.* 1996; 52: 3 – 11.

[39] Leone A. Biochemical markers of cardiovascular damage from tobacco smoke. *Curr. Pharm. Design.* 2005; 11: 2199 – 208.

[40] Schulte MA, Waller BF, Hull MT, Pless JE. Origin of the left anterior descending artery from the right aortic sinus with intramyocardial tunneling to the left side of the heart via the ventricular septum: A case against clinical and morphologic significance of myocardial bridging. *Am. Heart J.* 1985; 110: 499 – 501.

[41] Spach MS, Howell DA, Harris JS. Myocardial infarction and multiple thrombosis in a child with primary thrombocytosis. *Pediatrics.* 1963; 31: 268 – 76.

[42] Astrup P. The arterial wall in atherogenesis. In Cavallero ed., Atherogenesis, Padua, *Piccin Medical Book.* 1965; 77 – 92.

[43] Aird WC. Hemostasis and irreducible complexity. *J. Thromb. Haemost.* 2003; 1: 227 – 30.

[44] ten Cate H, Aird WC. Lessons from venous thrombosis and disseminated intravascular coagulation: a synthesis of pathophysiological mechanisms of pro-thrombotic states. In *Molecular Mechanisms of Disseminated Intravascular Coagulation,* tenCate H and Levi M eds., Landes Bioscience Publisher, Texas; 2003.

[45] Ross R. Atherosclerosis: an inflammation disease. *N. Engl. J. Med.* 1999; 340: 115 – 26.

[46] Celermajer DS, Adams MR, Clarkson P, Robinson J, McRedie R, Donald A, Deanfield JE. Passive smoking and impaired endothelium-dependent arterial dilatation in healthy young adults. *N. Engl. J. Med.* 1996; 334: 150 – 4.

[47] Pittilo RM, Mackie IJ, Rowles PM, Machine SJ, Woolf N. Effects of cigarette smoking on the ultrastructure of rat thoracic aorta, and its ability to produce prostacyclin. *Thromb. Haemost.* 1982; 48: 173 – 6.

[48] Davis J, Shelton L, Watanabe I, Arnold J. Passive smoking affects endothelium and platelets. *Arch. Intern. Med.* 1989; 149: 386 – 9.

[49] Sinzinger H, Kefalides A. Passive smoking severely decreases platelet sensitivity to antiaggregatory prostaglandins. *Lancet.* 1982; 2: 392 – 3.

[50] Burghuber O, Punzengruber C, Sinzinger H, Haber P, Silberbauer K. Platelet sensitivity to prostacyclin in smokers and non-smokers. *Chest.* 1986; 90: 34 – 8.

[51] Martin JF, Bath PM, Burr ML. Influence of platelet size on outcome after myocardial infarction. *Lancet.* 1991; 338: 1409 – 11.

[52] Stone MC, Thorpe JM. Plasma-fibrinogen- a major coronary risk factor. *JR. Coll. Gen. Pract.* 1985; 35: 565 – 9.

[53] Taddei S, Ghiadoni L, Virdis A, Versari D, Salvetti A. Mechanisms of endothelial dysfunction: clinical significance and preventive non-pharmacological therapeutic strategies. *Curr. Pharm. Design.* 2003; 9: 2385 – 402.

[54] Lusis AJ. Atherosclerosis. *Nature.* 2000; 407: 233 – 41.

[55] Libby P, Simon DI. Inflammation and thrombosis: the clot thickens. *Circulation.* 2001; 103: 1718 – 20.

[56] Prerovsky I, Hladovek J. Suppression of the desquamating effect of smoking on the human endothelium by hydroxyethylrutosides. *Blood Vessels.* 1979; 16: 239 – 40.

[57] Miyaura S, Eguchi H, Johnson JM. Effect of a cigarette smoke extract on the metabolism of the proinflammatory autacoid, platelet-activating factor. *Circ. Res.* 1992; 70: 341 – 7.

[58] Moreno PR, Purushothaman KR, Fuster V, Echeverri D, Truszczynska H, Sharma SK, Badimon JJ, O'Connor WN. Plaque neovascularization is increased in ruptured atherosclerotic lesions of human aorta: implications for plaque vulnerability. *Circulation.* 2004; 110: 2032 – 8.

[59] Luscher TF, Creager MA, Beckman JA, Cosentino F. Diabetes and vascular disease: pathophysiology, clinical consequences, and medical therapy. *Circulation.* 2003; 108: 1655 – 61.

[60] Kario K, Matsuo T, Kobayashi H. Which factors affect high D-dimer levels in the elderly? *Thromb. Res.* 1991; 62: 501 – 8.

[61] Salomaa V, Stinson V, Kark JD, Folsom AR, Davis CE, Wu KK. Association of fibrinolytic parameters with early atherosclerosis. The ARIC Study. Atherosclerosis risk in Communities Study. *Circulation.* 1995; 91: 284 – 90.

[62] Lassila R, Peltonen S, Lepantalo M, Saarinen O, Kauhanen P, Manninen V. Severity of peripheral atherosclerosis is associated with fibrinogen and degradation of cross-linked fibrin. *Arterioscler. Thromb.* 1993; 13: 1738 – 42.

[63] Herren T, Stricker H, Haeberli A, Do DD, Straub PW. Fibrin formation and degradation in patients with atherosclerotic disease. *Circulation.* 1994; 90: 2679 – 86.

[64] Smith FB, Rumley A, Lee AJ, Leng GC, Fowkes FG, Lowe GD. Haemostatic factors and prediction of ischaemic heart disease and stroke in claudicants. *Br. J. Haematol.* 1998; 100: 758 – 63.

[65] Hill D, Larcombe D, Refshauge J. Smoking and impairment of performance. *Med. J. Aust.* 1978; 2: 60 – 3.

[66] Anderson RF, Allensworth DC, DeGroot WJ. Myocardial toxicity from carbon monoxide poisoning: *Ann. Int. Med.* 1967; 1172 – 82.

[67] Marius-Nunez AL. Myocardial infarction with normal coronary arteries after acute exposure to carbon monoxide. *Chest.* 1990; 97: 491 – 4.

[68] Gvozdjakova A, Buda V, Sany L, Kurcharska J, Kruty F, Bozek P, Trstansky L, Gvozdjak J. Smoke cardiomyopathy: disturbance of oxidative processes in myocardial mitochondria. *Cardiovasc. Research.* 1984; 18: 229 – 32.

[69] Thomsen HK, Kjeldsen K. Threshold limit for carbon monoxide-induced myocardial damage. *Arch. Environ. Health.* 1974; 29: 73 – 8.

[70] Lough J. Cardiomyopathy produced by cigarette smoke. Ultrastructural observations in guinea pig. *Arch. Pathol. Lab. Med.* 1978; 102: 377 – 80.

[71] Kjeldsen K, Thomsen HK, Astrup P. Effects of carbon monoxide on myocardium. Ultrastructural changes in rabbits after moderate, chronic exposure. *Circ. Res.* 1974; 34: 339 – 48.
[72] Leone A, Bertanelli F, Mori L, Fabiano P, Battaglia A. Features of ischaemic cardiac pathology resulting from cigarette smoking. *J. Smoking-Related Dis.* 1994;5: 109 – 14.
[73] Leone A, Lopez M. Myocardial infarction and coronary damage in the smokers: histopathologic features. XII Inter-American Congress of Cardiology, Vancouver, Canada, 1985; 13 Abstract.
[74] Winniford MD, Jansen DE, Reynolds JA, Apprill P, Black WH, Hillis LD. Cigarette smoking-induced coronary vasoconstriction in atherosclerotic coronary artery disease and prevention by calcium antagonists and nitroglycerin. *Am. J. Cardiol.* 1987; 59: 203 – 7.
[75] Talks SJ, Chong NH, Gibson JM, Dodson PM. Fibrinogen, cholesterol and smoking as risk factors for non-arteritic anterior ischaemic optic neuropathy. *Eye.* 1995; 9: 85 – 8.
[76] Prentice RC, Carrol R, Scanlon PJ, Thomas JXJ. Recent exposure to cigarette smoke increases myocardial infarct size. *J. Am. Coll. Cardiol.* 1989; 13: 124A .
[77] Quillen JE, Rossen JD, Oskarsson HJ, Minor RLJ, Lopez AG, Winniford MD. Acute effect of cigarette smoking on the coronary circulation: constriction of epicardial and resistance vessels. *J. Am. Coll. Cardiol.* 1993; 22: 642 – 7.
[78] Health or Smoking. Follow-up Report of the Royal College of Physicians. Pitman Publishing, London 1983.
[79] Tsiara S, Elisaf M, Mikhailidis DP. Influence of smoking on predictors of vascular disease. *Angiology.* 2003; 54: 507 – 30.
[80] Cooper J, Douglas AS. Fibrinogen level as a predictor of mortality in survivors of myocardial infarction. *Fibrinolysis.* 1991; 5: 105 – 8.
[81] Resch KL, Ernst E, Matai A, Paulsen HF. Fibrinogen and viscosity as risk factors for subsequent cardiovascuar events in stroke survivors. *Ann. Intern. Med.* 1992; 117: 371 – 5.
[82] Zhu B, Parmley WW. Hemodinamic and vascular effects of active and passive smoking. *Am. Heart J.* 1995; 130: 1270 – 75.
[83] Klein LW, Pichard AD, Holt J, Smith H, Gorlin R, Teichholz LE. Effects of chronic tobacco smoking on coronary circulation. *J. Am. Coll. Cardiol.* 1983; 1: 421 – 6.
[84] Pohjola S, Siltanen P, Romo M. Five-year survival of 728 patients after acute myocardial infarction. *Br. Heart J.* 1980; 43: 176 – 83.
[85] Daly LE, Mulkahy R, Graham IM, Hickey N. Long-term effect on mortality of stopping smoking after unstable angina and myocardial infarction. *BMJ.* 1983; 287: 324 – 6.
[86] Jenkins CD, Zyzansky SJ, Rosenman RH. Risk of a new myocardial infarction in middleaged men with manifest coronary heart disease. *Circulation.* 1976; 53: 342 – 7.
[87] Vliestra RE, Kronmal RA, Oberman A. Stopping smoking improves survival in patients with angiographically-proven coronary artery disease. *Am. J. Cardiol.* 1982; 49: 984A.
[88] Consensus: Estrogen use and postmenopausal women. National Institutes of Health Consensus Development Conference Summary 1979; 2: 8. A consensus on the state of the heart as relates to risks and benefits.
[89] Mishell DR Jr. Contraception: In: De Groot LJ ed. , *Endocrinology,* Vol 3, Grune_ Stratton, New York 1979; 1435 – 50.

[90] Leone A, Lopez M. Role du tabac et de la contraception orale dans l'infarctus du myocarde de la femme. Description d'un cas. *Pathologica.* 1984 ; 76 : 493 – 8.
[91] Leone A, Lopez M. Oral contraception, ovarian disorders and tobacco in myocardial infarction of woman. *Pathologica.* 1986: 78: 237 – 42.
[92] Rosemberg L, Slone D, Shapiro S, Kaufman DW, Stolley PD, Miettinen OS. Noncontraceptive estrogens and myocardial infarction in young women. *JAMA.* 1980; 244: 339 – 42.
[93] Ross RK, Paganini-Hill A, Mack TM, Arthur M, Henderson BE. Menopausal oestrogen therapy and protection from death from ischaemic heart disease. *Lancet.* 1981; 1: 858 – 60.
[94] Chastre J. *Infarctus du myocarde: role du tabac et des contraceptives oraux.* Nouvelle Press Med. 1977 ; 12 : 1005.
[95] Vessey MP, McPherson K, Yeates D. Mortality in oral contraceptive users. *Lancet.* 1981; I: 549 – 50.
[96] Kurth T, Kase CS, Berger K, Graziano JM, Cook NR, Buring JE. Smoking and risk of hemorrhagic stroke in women. *Stroke.* 2003; 34: 2792 – 5.
[97] Hurn PD, Brass LM. Estrogen and stroke: a balanced analysis. *Stroke.* 2003; 34: 338 – 41.
[98] Higashi Y, Sanada M, Sasaki S, Nakagawa K, Goto C, Matsura H, Ohama K, Chayama K, Oshima T. Effect of estrogen replacement therapy on endothelial function in peripheral resistance arteries in normotensive and hypertensive postmenopausal women. *Hypertension.* 2001; 37: 651 – 7.
[99] Stier CT Jr, Chander PN, Rosenfeld L, Powers CA. Estrogen promotes microvascular pathology in female stroke-prone spontaneously hypertensive rats. *Am. J. Physiol. Endocrinol. Metab.* 2003; 285: E 232 – 9.
[100] Tsuda K, Kinoshita-Shimamoto Y, Mabuchi Y, Nishio I. Hormone replacement therapy improves membrane fluidity of erythrocytes in postmenopausal women: an electron paramagnetic resonance investigation. *Am. J. Hypertens.* 2003; 16: 502 – 7.
[101] Wassertheil-Smoller S, Hendrik SL, Limacher M, Heiss G, Kooperberg C, Baird A, Kotchen T, Curb DJ, Black H, Rossouw EJ, Aragaki A, Safford M, Stein E, MD, Laowattana S, Mysiw JW, for the WHI Investigators et al. Effect of estrogen plus progestin on stroke in postmenopausal women: the Women's Health Initiative: a randomized trial. *JAMA.* 2003; 289: 2673 – 84.
[102] Rexrode KM, Manson JE, Lee IM, Ridker PM, Sluss PM, Cook NR, Buring EJ. Sex hormone levels and risk of cardiovascular events in postmenopausal women. *Circulation.* 2003; 108: 1688 – 93.
[103] Humphrey LL, Chan BKS, Sox Jr. Postmenopausal hormone replacement therapy and the primary prevention of cardiovascular disease. *Ann. Intern. Med.* 2002; 137 (4): 273 – 84.
[104] Miller J, Chan BKS, Nelson HD. Hormone replacement therapy and risk of venous thromboembolism: a systematic review and meta-analysis. *Ann. Intern. Med.* 2002; 136 (3): 680 – 90.
[105] Wilson PW, Garrison RJ, Castelli WP. Postmenopausal estrogen use, cigarette smoking, and cardiovascular morbidity in women over 50. The Framingham Study. *N. Engl. J. Med.* 1985; 313 (17): 1038 – 43.

[106] Petitti DB, Perlman JA, Sidney S. Non contraceptive estrogens and mortality: long-term follow-up of women in the Walnut Creek Study. *Obstet Gynecol.* 1987; 70: 289 – 93.

[107] Mueck AO, Seeger H. Smoking, estradiol metabolism, and hormone replacement therapy. *Arzneimittelforschung.* 2003; 53: 1 – 11.

[108] Tsuda K, Nishio I. A selective estrogen receptor modulator, tamoxifen, and membrane fluidity of erythrocytes in normotensive and hypertensive postmenopausal women: an Electron Paramagnetic Resonance investigation. *AJH.* 2005; 18: 1067 – 76.

[109] Gotto AM Jr, Brinton EA. Assessing low levels of high density lipoprotein cholesterol as a risk factor in coronary heart disease: a working group report and update. *J. Am. Coll. Cardiol.* 2004; 43: 717 – 24.

[110] Havel RJ, Kane JP. Structure and metabolism of plasma lipoproteins. In: Scriver CR, Beaudet AL, Sly WS, Valle D eds. The Metabolic and Molecular Bases of Inherited Disease II, 7th ed, Mc-Graw-Hill, New York 1995; 1841 – 51.

[111] Azizi F, Raiszadeh F, Salehi P, Rahmani M, Emami H, Ganbarian A, Hajipour R. Determinanants of serum HDL-C level in a Tehran urban population: the Tehran Lipid and Glucose Study. *Nutr. Metab. Cardiovasc. Dis.* 2002;12: 80 – 9.

[112] Mizoue T, Ueda R, Hino Y, Yoshimura T. Workplace exposure to environmental tobacco smoke and high density lipoprotein cholesterol among nonsmokers. *Am. J. Epidemiol.* 1999; 150: 1068 – 72.

[113] Moffat RJ, Stamford BA, Biggerstaff KD. Influence of worksite environmental tobacco smoke on serum lipoprotein profiles of female non-smokers. *Metabolism.* 1995; 44: 1536 – 9.

[114] Moffat RJ, Chelland SA, Pecott DL, Stamford BA. Acute exposure to environmental tobacco smoke reduces HDL-C and HDL2-C. Preventive Medicine 2004; 38: 637 – 41.

[115] Kwiterovich PO Jr. The antiatherogenic role of high-density lipoprotein cholesterol. *Am. J. Cardiol.* 1998; 82: 13Q – 21Q.

[116] Tall AR. An overview of reverse cholesterol transport. *European Heart Journal.* 1998; 19: A31 – 5.

[117] Moskowitz W, Mosteller M, Schieken R, Bossano R, Hewitt J, Bodurtha J, Segrest J. Lipoprotein and oxygen transport alterations in passive smoking preadolescent children: the MCV Twin study. *Circulation.* 1990; 81: 586 – 92.

[118] Neufeld EJ, Mictus-Snyder M, Beiser AS, Baker AL, Newburger JW. Passive cigarette smoking and reduced HDL-Cholesterol levels in children with high-risk lipid profiles. *Circulation.* 1997; 96: 1403 – 7.

[119] Feldman J, Shenker IR, Etzel RA, Spierto FW, Liliefield DE, Nussbaum M, Jacobson MS. Passive smoking alters lipid profiles in adolescents. *Pediatrics.* 1991;88:259 – 64.

[120] Rimm EB, Can J, Stampfer MJ, Colditz GA, Willet WC. Prospective study of cigarette smoking, alcohol use, and the risk of diabetes in men. *BMJ.* 1995; 310: 555 – 9.

[121] Wannamethee SG, Shaper AG, Perry IJ. Smoking as a modifiable risk factor for type 2 diabetes in middle-aged men. *Diabetes Care.* 2001; 24: 1590 – 5.

[122] Rimm EB, Manson JE, Stampfer MJ, Colditz GA, Willet WC, Rosner B, Hennekens CH, Speizer FE. Cigarette smoking and the risk of diabetes in women. *Am. J. Public Health.* 1993; 83: 211 – 4.

[123] Kawakami N, Takatsuka N, Shimizu H, Ishibashi H. Effects of smoking on the incidence of non-insulin-dependent diabetes mellitus: replication and extension in a Japanese cohort of male employees. *Am. J. Epidemiol.* 1997; 145: 103 – 9.

[124] Haire-Joshu D, Glasgow RE, Tibbs TL. Smoking and diabetes. *Diabetes Care.* 1999; 22: 1887 – 98.

[125] Houston TK, Person SD, Pletcher MJ, Liu K, Iribarren C, Kiefe CI. Active and passive smoking and development of glucose intolerance among young adults in a prospective cohort: CARDIA study. *BMJ.* 2006; 332: 1064 – 9.

[126] Kendall DM, Sobel BE, Coulston AM, Peters-Harmel AL, McLean BK, Peregallo-Dittko V, Buse JB, Fonseca VA, Hill JO, Nesto RW, Sunyer FX. The insulin resistance syndrome and coronary artery disease. *Coron Artery Dis.* 2003; 14: 335 – 48.

[127] Reaven GM. The insulin resistance syndrome: Definition and dietary approaches to treatment. *Annu. Rev. Nutr.* 2005; 25: 391 – 406.

[128] Henkin L, Zaccaro D, Haffner S, Karter A, Rewers M, Sholinsky P, Wagenknecht L. Cigarette smoking, environmental tobacco smoke exposure and insulin sensitivity: the Insulin Resistance Atherosclerosis Study. *Ann. Epidemiol.* 1999; 9: 290 – 6.

[129] Reaven GM, Tsao PS. Insulin resistance and compensatory hyperinsulinemia: the key player between cigarette smoking and cardiovascular disease? *J. Am. Coll. Cardiol.* 2003; 41: 1044 – 7.

[130] Block G, Dietrich M, Norkus EP, Morrow JD, Hudes M, Caan B, Packer L. Factors associated with oxidative stress in human populations. *Am. J. Epidemiol.* 2002; 156: 274 – 85.

[131] Harrison D, Griendling KK, Landmesser U, Hornig B, Drexler H. Role of oxidative stress in atherosclerosis. *Am. J. Cardiol.* 2003; 91: 7A – 11A.

[132] Kosecik M, Erel O, Sevinc E, Selek S. Increased oxidative stress in children exposed to passive smoking. *Int. J. Cardiol.* 2005; 100: 61 – 4.

[133] Haskell WL. *Primer in Preventive Cardiology.* In: Pearson TA, Criqui MH, Luepker RW, Oberman A, Winston M eds. American Heart Association, Dallas, 1994; 173 – 87.

[134] Schectman G, Byrd JC, Gruchow HW. The influence of smoking on vitamin C status in adults. *Am. J. Public Health.* 1989; 79: 158 – 62.

[135] Heitzer T, Just H, Munzel T. Antioxidant vitamin C improves endothelial dysfunction in chronic smokers. *Circulation.* 1996; 94: 6 – 9.

[136] Rimm EB, Stampfer MJ, Ascherio A, Giovannucci E, Colditz GA, Willet WC. Vitamin E consumption and the risk of coronary heart disease in men. *N. Engl. J. Med.* 1993; 328: 1450 – 6.

[137] The Alpha-Tocopherol, Beta Carotene Cancer Prevention Study Group. The effect of vitamin E and beta carotene on the incidence of lung cancer and other cancers in male smokers. *N. Engl. J. Med.* 1994; 330: 1029 – 35.

[138] Neunteufl T, Priglinger U, Heher S, Zehetgruber M, Soregi G, Lehr S, Huber K, Maurer G, Weidinger F, Kostner K. Effects of vitamin E on chronic and acute endothelial dysfunction in smokers. *J. Am. Coll. Cardiol.* 2000; 35: 277 – 83.

Chapter 7

STATISTICS FOR UNDERSTANDING DAMAGE

ABSTRACT

Statistical methods used to assess cardiovascular damage derived from passive smoking exposure should be formulated carefully by experts in statistics but not anyone of researchers since many variables may interfere with conducted studies.

An analysis of the significance of the main statistical parameters – statistical certainty and probability, percentage and mean values, confidence interval, relative risk in observational studies, chi-squared tests (χ^2), p value – is briefly conducted in an attempt to establish the role of statistics in the studies on passive smoking exposure.

Moreover, metanalysis, a statistical method whereby all data from all available findings on the same subject are combined to assess the significance of a phenomenon, explains what concerns passive smoking.

Finally, obtained results on cardiovascular damage from passive smoking should be estimated carefully since some statistical limits may exist. The most important limits are an incorrect estimate of mathematical level of the p value, a wrong drawing of the study, limited duration of the same, health status of study population who can have associated other cardiovascular risk factors that potentiate the damage attributed fully to passive smoking in the wrong way.

Keywords: Passive smoking, statistics, statistical certainty, statistical probability, mean, percentage, confidence interval, risk, relative risk, chi-squared test(s), p value.

The large majority of data that identify passive smoking exposure as a risk factor for cardiovascular system come from epidemiological findings conducted on populations who were different in demographics, lifestyle, race, sex, age, socio-economic status and many other characteristics, although the great number of individuals included in the study sample can lead to conclusions having – in the cases of similar responses – a statistical validation. Therefore, obtained observations must be analyzed and then estimated by those mathematical models which led to results of an almost similar comparison.

Statistics and epidemiology must be recognized as basic sciences to promote public health. Together, they provide significant information for understanding the outcome and prognosis of a disease and therefore permit to build effective measures of preventive medicine.

Epidemiology contributes either to the knowledge of the distribution and prevailing of a disease or to evaluate where better health conditions exist or how to reach both these objectives. Therefore, primary purpose of the epidemiology is to search for those factors, favoring the appearance of a disease and avoiding their negative effects. That is possible to be obtained only by large-scale findings on the studied subject.

Statistical methodologies permit to establish those factors that epidemiologic findings attribute to be related to the appearance of a specific disease which are really factors of risk since they accompany the disease with a wider rate although not constantly. Therefore, statistical methods [1] play a vital role in control of health status and also permit to understand if the estimate of a specific characteristic is a manifestation of primary importance. Statistical methodologies are widely used to monitor different factors according to the characteristics of the studied disease and make these factors valid with statements of confidence related to their estimates. By doing so, every type of studies, clinical studies, experimental studies and many others, can be drawn in a manner that a maximum amount of data can be obtained and consequently, a more effective approach to the characteristics of a specific disease carried out. However, there exists the probability that an incorrect analysis of statistical methods [2–4] can reach unreliable results. Another important aspect of statistical methods is to reach a clearly numerical presentation of the results as well as their correct interpretation. Incorrect interpretations of the results can lead to erroneous conclusions. Fortunately, the progresses in the study of statistical methodology tend to reduce incorrect interpretations, although some limits are particularly recognized in collecting material which depends widely from interpretation, that could vary, of single researchers engaged in the same research. Unfortunately, nowadays, epidemiological studies are large-scale studies with populations enrolled in different centers and also countries. Therefore, statistical studies can provide effective data on the characteristics of a phenomenon even if they often fail to reproduce it exactly for the whole studied populations. Moreover, recording too much information as a purpose of statistical studies on large-scale often leads to confusion in evaluating the results with care [5].

Reproducibility of almost similar results must be the objective of a finding, in order to remove not unanimous opinions. These conditions are mainly obtained in experimental rather than large scale-studies.

Beyond every debate, however, statistics provides effective information on a studied sample on condition that one can interpret correctly the statistical certainty and probability theory to understand the applied methodologies as well as their reliability.

A statistical method therefore, if correctly applied, permits to verify the certainty, different degree of probability of a hypothesis, but also the total invalidity of the same hypothesis that, in the latter condition, should be rejected. Such a knowledge is basic for what concerns the epidemiological findings on cardiovascular damage from passive smoking exposure, since a unanimous interpretation of damage does not exist particularly because of a lack of a constant reproducibility of the same results. Indeed, they have been particularly obtained from large-scale epidemiological studies.

STATISTICAL CERTAINTY AND PROBABILITY

The concept of the theory of certainty and probability plays an unchangeable role for an exact estimate and validation of the methodologies of an epidemiological study, particularly large-scale studies [6–8] under a statistical profile.

Certainty is a statistical condition where an event has a probability of occurrence equal to 1 (100%), therefore, there is evidence of an indisputable proof. The estimate of this parameter provides for the presence of two types of events: events with positive response (pr) and total of possible events (p). Ratio (C) between the first parameter and second parameter denotes statistical value of certainty when the two events are equal in number:

$$C = \frac{pr}{p}$$

The value of C, being a ratio between the number of observations with positive responses and the number of all possible observations can vary from 0 to 1. C = 0 is when pr is = 0; therefore, there is no possibility. On the contrary, if we can observe all events to have positive response, the C value will be equal to 1 (100 % of responses).

C = 1 therefore, is a value that denotes mathematically full statistical significance of the analyzed parameter.

On the contrary, probability is a measure of the relative frequency or likelihood of the occurrence of an event. Values are derived from a theoretical distribution or more frequently, from clinical or experimental observations with positive response and/or negative response or no response. As one can see, in this case, there is no certainty. Therefore, if the percent of positive responses involve a large majority of analyzed observations and C is approximately nearest to 1, the observed events have a statistically significant value, but not the absolute certainty. Statistical significance will be better described later in this chapter.

To better understand this basic concept and therefore to attribute a statistical significance of a different degree in a study design, it is worthwhile to apply to the example of the two balls with different colour: for an example, one white ball and one black ball.

Putting the two balls into a bag and then pulling out, at random, one of the balls, only two possibilities exist: one can pull out the white ball or the black ball with no knowledge of the colour that firstly will appear. Really, statistical hypothesis can be formulated as follows:

½ (white ball) + ½ (black ball) = 2/2 = 1 (total balls)

and number 1 satisfies the two possible measures.

In the case of pulling a small number, but different from one, there exists the possibility that one colour ball can casually exceed the other colour, even if in a very little amount. Statistically, this possibility is considered to characterize observations until 1 to 100.

If the greatest number of pullings occur, the matter completely changes. The two colours must be equal or almost equal in the number of pullings out to have a strong certainty (C) of a statistically significant result. If pulling out is repeated more and more times and always a colour prevails on the other several times, such a fact means that there are known or unknown factors not related to pulling out as itself but, strictly influencing pulling out itself and, moreover, capable to influence the phenomenon. Therefore, C would exist only in case of knowledge of all those factors which interfere with the phenomenon and such a matter, as one can intuit, is far to be realized. An agreement needs to be reached for interpreting the results of the phenomenon. Mathematical measures provided by statistics contribute to that.

Some statistical concepts must be formulated. After the estimate of sample size and characteristic, establishing all those quantitative data (data which are expressed by numerical values) or qualitative data (data which are classified by type but not by number) would be an effective method to initiate a statistical process. Before assessing arithmetic mean (average of data to be analyzed) or median (the middle value in a distribution, below and above which values with equal total frequencies or probabilities lie), and standard deviation (measure of spread or dispersion. It is root mean square deviation) or standard error (the standard deviation of the means of samples of given size drawn from examined data), it should be important, in my opinion, to evaluate and classify all conditioning events – those events which are known to have occured or the probability that another not well estimated event may occur – of the statistical process.

That is better particularly in findings concerning environmental tobacco smoke exposure, since the environment characteristics may strongly influence cardiovascular damage from smoking and, therefore, the analysis of all possible conditioning events that can be related to the exposure may provide more reliable results.

PERCENTAGE VALUE, MEAN VALUES AND CONFIDENCE INTERVAL

Statistical analysis provides a number limited of estimates of a phenomenon or characteristics in a group of population that is to be considered a statistical sample. Purpose of the estimates is, however, to extend the values of an estimated parameter from the statistical sample to all population from where the sample comes. Theoretically, studied population could be characterized by the largest unknown number of individuals as well as lifestyle habits. Therefore, there is need to know how collected data of the analyzed phenomenon can be translated to the entire population as well as to estimate that the procedures of translation are correctly conducted.

Estimate of the above concept needs to establish the frequency of a distribution calculated as percentage of the whole sample as a first step. Therefore, the percent number of observations related to studied parameters can be calculated by ratio:

$$\% R = f/n$$

where %R is the ratio between the frequency of the phenomenon (f= frequency) and total number (n) of the sample. Percentage is a proportion per hundred parts. To know the true value of a percentage, it is basic to estimate the limits within which changes of percentage could be due to chance. Assessing the confidence interval can help to solve this problem.

Confidence interval is that interval within which a studied parameter is calculated, according to the data of the sample, to establish if probability of lying exists. It is very important to keep in mind that the larger the sample size, the smaller the confidence interval.

When a value of a phenomenon falls within the confidence interval one can conclude that it is precise with a strong frequency. The 95% confidence interval means that there is a probability of 95% that the percentage of an estimated parameter is true. 99% confidence interval identifies a 99% of probability, and so on. As aforesaid above, statistical values not related to chance must belong to a larger sample and meet conventionally confidence interval measures of, at least, 95%.

Some observations on the harmful effects of passive smoking exposure show measures that are, epidemiologically, a little out on the confidence interval, whereas a large majority of findings meets those characteristics of width of the studied sample that permit a significant statistical interpretation with probabilities that are lying from 95% confidence interval and over.

Mean values of comparison of different parameters have less importance for statistically establishing damage related to passive smoking exposure.

Mathematical formulae to numerically calculate the discussed parameters are not a purpose of this issue that set only the knowledge of the main principles that regulate statistical responses of epidemiological studies related to passive smoking exposure. They can be found easily in each statistics book [6–8].

The Risk in Observational Studies

When we analyze the negative effects of smoking exposure on individuals, primarily we must face the degree of risk of those populations who are exposed as well as the reasons of the prevailing negative effects on some individuals rather than others. Therefore, firstly, one needs to establish if there is evidence of a statistically significant association of a specific event with that risk factor, specifically passive smoking exposure. Therefore, one must be capable to correctly interpret the types of studies that may be conducted.

There are three types of observational studies (Table 7.1.): case-control studies, transversal studies, and cohort studies.

Case-control studies are conducted on two groups of subjects, the one clearly showing manifestations of a negative event, the other with no manifestation. Then, one analyzes which group of subjects usually met the negative event. Clear examples of case-control studies are epidemiological studies related to risk factors, and among them, particularly smoking, since it is a factor that theoretically could be avoided.

Transversal studies are conducted on those populations affected by the manifestations of a negative event as well as the exposure to analyze harmful factor. Collected data concern current epidemiological observations, often those hypothesized but not fully known conclusions.

The third type of study – cohort studies – concerns populations that are not yet affected by a negative event. Then, characteristics of the negative event should be established. Findings follow the future course of those phenomena related to both studied populations and event.

Table 7.1. Types of observational studies and their characteristics

Type of study	Characteristic
1. Case-control study	Relationship between population exposed in the past to a negative event and its effects.
2. Transversal study	Current epidemiological data provided by a direct observation between obtained results and studied event.
3. Cohort study	Prospective analysis on the possible relation between a negative event and exposed people.

Each type of observational studies provide two basic data: the number of subject sample affected negatively by passive smoking exposure and the percentage of the total. These two parameters permit to calculate those measures (chi-squared, p-value) of statistical significance that will be described ahead.

Described concepts to evaluating a statistical significance of a phenomenon, particularly smoking, can be estimated by an example derived from the data of a previous study [9].

Well, let's analyze the response of a total number of 1,432 subjects, partly exposed to smoking- current smokers - (1,232 subjects) and 200 never smokers. Therefore, smoking exposure was the negative event. Hypertension was the study parameter related to exposure or non-exposure in 774 people (100% of hypertensive patients), so that there were 700 hypertensive subjects (90 %) who had been exposed to smoking and damaged by smoking itself and 74 (10 %) without negative effects of smoking. Of a total number of 658 patients without hypertension, 532 patients (81 %) had been exposed to smoking, whereas the other 126 (19%) did not suffer from the negative effects of smoking. The question is: are there negative effects of smoking for both groups, hypertensive patients and patients without hypertension, or for only one group, hypertensive patients or patients without hypertension?

According to statistical methodology, a table containing numerically four characteristics, two for examined subjects and two for each event, may be built (Table 7.2.).

Table 7.2. Table of the risk for studied patients

Patients	Negative effect (smoking)	No negative effect	Total
Hypertensive people	700 (A)	74 (C)	774 (A+ C)
Non hypertensive patients	532 (B)	126 (D)	658 (B + D)
Total	1,232 (A + B)	200 (C + D)	1,432 (A+B+C+D)
RR (relative risk) = 1.54			

There is now the possibility to calculate the proportional relationship between subjects affected or unaffected by smoking according to their clinical characteristic, namely presence or absence of hypertension, since the Table 7.2 display numerical values and therefore quantitative parameters.

Proportionally, hypertensive patients affected by smoking will be:

$$A/ (A+C) = 700/ (700 + 74) = 0.9 = 90\%$$

Nonhypertensive patients affected by smoking must be, if statistical distribution is true, 10 percent; by the formula:

B / (B + D) = 532 / (532 + 126) = 0.8

(that, because numerical gap, will be in rounding 1 = 10%).

As it can be seen, there are corresponding percentage values and therefore the degree of risk may be calculated. In Table 7.2, there is evidence of a strong relationship between smoking and hypertension: the risk of appearance of hypertension for a smoker is one and a half times more frequent than in never smokers. Moreover, such a statement well correlated a chi-squared (χ^2) value calculated of 26.419 that coincides with a p statistically highly significant. From these observations, it can be noted that a new statistical parameter has been introduced: the chi-squared test (χ^2) that is widely applied for establishing statistical estimates.

Statistical knowledge of those parameters that characterize an event is basic to estimate statistical significance that usually crosses t-student test of comparison by calculating, precisely, χ^2 and p value that expresses conventionally the measure of significance.

Chi-Squared (χ^2) Tests

In an attempt to clarify the estimate of the test χ^2 , χ^2 distribution needs to be discussed. The latter parameter is used in a large number of statistical tests including the χ^2 test. It is the distribution with n degrees of freedom of $X^2_1 + X^2_{\bar{1}} \ldots + X^2_n$, where X (1, $\bar{1}$, n) are n independent normal random variables with mean 0 and variance 1.

Chi-squared- test (χ^2) is used to measure how well a set of observations meets a particular discrete distribution. If the theoretical distribution shows that value X_1 must occur an expected number of times, named E_i, but it really occurs O_i times, that is the true number of times, chi-squared will be:

$$\chi^2 = \sum_{i \approx 1} \frac{(O_i - E_i)^2}{E_i}$$

where:

O_i is an observed frequency
E_i is an expected theoretical frequency

Then, there will be a chi-squared distribution with n – p degrees of freedom, where p is the number of distribution parameters used in calculating E_i.

Therefore, if χ^2 is large, the hypothetical distribution should be rejected. So, we are able to understand the concept of invalidity of a formulated hypothesis and then, the logical conclusion that it may be rejected.

The test can be used to estimate a continuous distribution by collecting data, but a careful collecting must be conducted to avoid dubious results and therefore, arbitrary interpretation of the data. The above formulae permit to calculate theoretically the values of estimated data. To obtain a quantitative and effective measure of the significance of the event, alphabetical letters used to explain the above formulae must be replaced by respective mathematical numbers provided by the event under study.

There are some limits in applying the mathematical calculus. Indeed, if several of E_i values are smaller than about 5, the test cannot be used unless changes are given. However, this occurence does not concern epidemiological parameters as well as the number of subjects exposed to passive smoking, being these findings are usually conducted on a great amount of observations.

Among the different chi-squared tests, t-test, or Student's t-test, is a test used on the means of small samples and may follow two ways. Firstly, the sample has been drawn from a population of a given mean and unknown standard deviation that must be calculated from the sample. Secondly, two samples have both been drawn from the same population and statistically possible differences about the two samples must be established. Therefore, the t-test estimates whether the means of two groups belonging to the same population, but had undergone an event with a different response, are statistically different from each to other. There is a study group and a control group, and the ratio between the differences for the studied parameter in the two groups divided for the group variables provide statistical estimate of a t-test.

On the contrary, Pearson's chi-square test is one of a variety of chi-square tests, namely those statistical procedures of the results of which are evaluated by reference to the chi-square distribution [10]. The purpose of the test is to verify if the relative frequences that meet a specific event follow a particular frequency of distribution. The analyzed event is estimated to be independent and have the same characteristics of distribution.

Pearson's χ^2-test is used to assess two types of comparison: test of goodness of fit and test of independence. The first test evaluates whether or not an observed frequency distribution deviates from the theoretical distribution. The second type of test verifies if paired observations related to two variables are independent from eachother.

Usually, Pearson's t-test is used in the event of large number samples, whereas student's t-test find it being applied in smaller, but statistically enough, study samples. Frequently, paired t-test use may be seen particularly in experimental observations as experimental findings on passive smoking exposure where the number of included people is, of course, smaller than that of large-scale observational studies.

P Value

The statistical significance of an estimate depends on the probability that the observed variables or differences in a study sample could occur merely by chance or otherwise, through a strong relationship among different parameters of the sample. On the first event, there is no statistical link between study population and analyzed phenomenon – it can be said that the phenomenon is a pure consequence of the chance with no statistically relationship. On the second instance, study phenomenon is related to the statistical estimate and then, there is evidence of significance in the examined parameters. P value is the expression of a statistical or not significant value, according to its percent value.

Let's see the reasons of that.

Usually, statistical significance of an observation establishes the degree of truth as well as representative level of observation itself.

Specifically, the p value is the probability of error that can be allowed in accepting our studied data as valid results. Particularly, apvaluelessthan0.05has a statistically "conventional" significance in observed results since it means that there is less than 5 percent of probability that the relationship between studied variables of the examined sample has occurred by chance. Ofcourse, a p value less than 0.01 reduces the probability of the chance to 1 percent as well as smaller p values, therefore, affecting the level of statistical certainty. Moreover, in different types of research, particularly experimental findings, the p value with a statistical significance is customarily fixed at a level of p less than 0.05.

Then, a question arises: how to assess that a studied parameter has really a statistical significance and why a p value less than 0.05 can be used as a border-line statistical level by many researchers?

There are several factors that can clarify the above questions as well as determine the role of p value among the different statistical methodologies.

Assessing p value significance is related to observations which seem to show that if the probability of an event is higher, numerically, than 1/5, the event must be rejected, whereas if it is lower than 1/5, the appearance of the event could have a statistical significance. Such a statement is on arbitrarily conventional estimate that may be supported by the evidence that medical observations collected year after year, and for a long time, see that a relatinship between two specific phenomena could be most often associated.

The truthfulness of the facts is that the p value estimates a parameter of probability but not certainty. Certainty should exist only in the presence of a correlation of studied phenomena equal to 100 percent with then a p value = 0. Statistically, that is impossible. Therefore, attention should be set to those numbers of the p value that more close to 0, such as p less than 0.01,or better yet 0.001, or 0.0001, and so on. Moreover, there is evidence that a statistically significant result is not always related to a clinical or experimental positive outcome. Indeed, statistical significance of an event can lead, sometimes, to results without any benefits. A drug that reduces the LDL-Cholesterol of 1 mg/dl in a total population with elevated concentrations of the metabolite has the strongest statistical significance, but clinical effects are almost worthless. Therefore, a p value with a high statistical significance may be related to results that do not reach the expectation.

An analysis of those errors that we can meet in assessing the p value needs to be conducted to warrant the best result of the estimates. The main errors are listed in table 7.3.

Some of these are related to the characteristics of the study sample, some to researchers, and some more to obtained results and type of statistical methods that has been used. Avoiding these errors is basic to be in a position to assess whether the scientific effectiveness of a finding, especially of those findings where lifestyles or individual characteristics associated with the environment, race, or particularly harmful risk factors must be really maintained under control in an attempt to reduce their negative effects with undoubted improvement of individuals' health.

Table 7.3. Main errors met in assessing p value in statistical studies

1. Errors in the study sample	Sample numerically small
	Sample not homogenous
	Arbitrary enrollment
2. Errors to attribute to researchers	Excessive enthusiasm
	Excessive prudence
3. Errors in results and methods	Pointlessness of the result
	Not suitable method
	Incomplete study parameters

Thus, there could be the possibility that we emphasize - by an incorrect analysis of the p value - a result that really does not exist or, otherwise, the lack of a proven result.

Errors found in studies related to the negative effects of passive smoking exposure on cardiovascular system particularly concern the representative character of the sample used for the experimental finding (usually numerically small samples) as well as an excessive enthusiasm of some researchers, who are often longing to demonstrate a non-demonstrated idea, kept in their mind, that negative effects caused by passive smoking exposure really exist, and a statistical validation would be simply a surplus. That could further explain their reasons of establishing a p value less than 0.05 and more than 0.01, or higher, as statistically significant.

METANALYSIS

A large series of both epidemiological and experimental studies focused their attention on the same subject of research although they reached different results and conclusions. Such occurrences did not permit to assess the "real" value of the data of the examined experiments, resulting in much confusion to interpret them.

Although this observation may be revealed useful to interpret prudentially, the numerous aspects which characterize several problems in medicine, it can nevertheless cause a limited progress in our knowledge. Indeed, it does not provide information that may "help" to solve many questions, especially those where doubts on the cause-effect relationship of a phenomenon exist. All observed data, positive data and negative data, on the same research subject, may be combined by using metanalysis.

Metanalysis is a current statistical methodology whereby all data from all (or a possible maximum number) available findings on the same subject are combined, sometimes without care for the quality of the data, to better assess statistical significance of a phenomenon. Nowadays, metanalysis is widely used to get a maximum amount of statistical comparison, without worrying about possible distortion of the results. Thus, basic metanalysis tends only to enlarge the number of populations included in similar studies. By doing so, it is possible to verify the response to an event in a number of subjects much more statistically representative and then attribute a major value to the formulated hypothesis of the study as well as its conclusions.

Cardiovascular damage from passive smoking exposure has been assessed, among other things, by meta-analyses in some excellent papers of Wells [11] and Law and coworkers [12-13]. These studies included a different number of findings and, totally evaluated, they reached the conclusion that never smokers undergone passive smoking exposure had an impairment in cardiovascular responses.

It is not the purpose of this chapter to describe the characteristics of the metanalysis in detail. In my opinion, it is basic to know the principles that regulate this statistical methodology since it is used for increasing numerically the study sample. However, for findings by metanalysis when the different study populations are numerically raised, statistical methods used for assessing are the same as already described.

How Statistics Faces up Passive Smoking Findings

Statistics reach a "delicate" matter in estimating the negative effects caused by passive smoking exposure on cardiovascular system as they are published in the papers on the subject. Really, problems associated with tobacco industries, workplaces, home, and type of exposure to environmental tobacco smoke can lead, from time to time, to underestimate or overestimate the harmful effects of the phenomenon. Consequently, as it has been clarified above, statistical methods provide data of different degree of probability of a studied event but not certainty. Therefore, there is evidence that facing the different estimates that can be inferred by the analysis of the reports on the subject requires the attention and authority of specialists in this field. Avoiding misinterpretation of the results is the first and basic concept to establish the reliability of reached conclusions.

As aforesaid, statistical estimates have a different degree of significance with regard to their mathematical value. A p value generally less than 0.05 has much more probability to undergo a statistical error of significance rather than a p value less than 0.001. Therefore, the number that characterizes a p value is an incontrovertible fact to be considered when results on the negative effects derived from passive smoking exposure are analyzed.

The drawing of the study is not a less important factor. Studies derived from a direct observation and applying the protocol are certainly more valid than those findings derived from questionnaires – and there are a lot concerning the negative effects of passive smoking exposure, since the researcher, is personally devoted to conduct the study. Our unpublished observations [14] revealed that the questionnaires were not fully reliable. Indeed, we sent the same questionnaire twice to a number of subjects by affirming that their first answers to questionnaire had been lost. Well, different answers to the same question were provided, in a few cases, by the same people.

Moreover, the duration of the study is another parameter that a statistical estimate ought to include among the factors that are carefully considered. Really, there is a prolonged interval between exposure to passive smoking and occurence of those structural events that are the result of the damage, unless for certain experimental conditions where negative changes caused by smoking exposure are usually transient and therefore, hard to interpret correctly once the experiment has occurred.

Unfortunately, all aforesaid factors are not equal in several findings which are related to cardiovascular damage from passive smoking. Therefore, each statistical estimate should be conducted finding by finding and then equal parameters deriving from different protocols of study compared. Such a behavior could give better results for establishing the degree of damage.

Yet the health status of studied populations should be almost similar to avoid negative responses, which could be evaluated as a consequence of smoking exposure, which are really the results of other risk factors. Lacking knowledge of associated risk factors, particularly for those findings conducted by questionnaires, occurs in some studies where the conclusions are attributed to the whole study populations – subjects having or lacking associated risk factors.

From the analysis of all these possibilities, there emerge statistical methods to be used for a correct assessment of the damage from passive smoking exposure that should be drawn by experts in statistics but not assigned generally to just anyone of the researchers. Unfortunately, this is a limit in different fields of the statistics and represents a negative factor, particularly in the findings related to passive smoking where a large number of factors may interfere.

Going so far as to conclude, let's go back to the example of the two balls, black ball and white ball to interpret correctly the statistical significance of the damage due to smoking exposure. Figuratively we are in front of two events: people damaged by passive smoking exposure (black ball), and non-exposed people (white ball). As it can be seen, there are two possibilities of pulling out from the bag, black or white ball. There is evidence that the black ball would be pulled out more and more times in the large majority of cases, as a consequence of the fact that passive smoking exposure is that event that determines such a condition. Therefore, a statistically correct interpretation of the event is basic to approach, with a maximum of probability, statistical certainty and then fully estimate the significance of a damage.

Epidemiological findings conducted either clinically or experimentally on cardiovascular damage caused by passive smoking exposure do not always follows such a way. This is the main reason that explains the lack of unanimous opinions of some researchers on cardiovascular damage caused from passive smoking, lacking also the exact reproducibility of the damage on clinical reports. However, experimental findings [15] demonstrate carefully that cardiovascular damage derived from smoking exposure can be exactly reproduced when similar experimental procedures are used.

References

[1] Woodall WH. Controversies and contradictions in statistical process control. *Journal of Quality Technology*. 2000; 4: 341 – 50.

[2] Schor S, Karten I. Statistical evaluation of medical journal manuscripts. *JAMA*. 1966; 195: 1123 – 8.

[3] Gore SM, Jones IG, Rytter EC. Misuse of statistical methods: critical assessment of articles in BMJ from January to March 1976. *BMJ*. 1977; i: 85 – 7.

[4] White SJ. Statistical errors in papers in the British Journal of Psychiatry. *Br. J. Psychiatry*. 1979; 135: 336 – 42.

[5] Wright P, Haybittle J. Design of forms for clinical trials. *BMJ.* 1979; ii: 650 – 1.

[6] Glantz SA. *Primer of Biostatistics.* McGraw-Hill, New York, 1992.

[7] Porkess R. The Harper Collins Dictionary of Statistics. Harper Perennial, a Division of Harper Collins Publishers, New York, 1991.

[8] Geller S. Abrégé de Statistique. *Masson,* Paris 1983.

[9] Leone A, Lopez M, Picerno G. Il ruolo del fumo nel determinismo della cardiopatia coronarica. Ipotesi sul possibile meccanismo di danno miocardico. *Min. Cardioang.* 1984; 32: 435 – 9.

[10] Chernoff H, Lehmann EL. The use of maximum likelihood estimates in χ^2 tests for goodness-of-fit. *The Annals of Mathematical Statistics.* 1954; 25: 579 – 86.

[11] Wells AJ. Passive smoking as a cause of heart disease. *J. Am. Coll. Cardiol.* 1994; 24: 546 – 54.

[12] Law MR, Hackshaw AK. Environmental tobacco smoke. *Br. Med. Bull.* 1996; 52: 22 – 34.

[13] Law MR, Morris JK, Wald NJ. Environmental tobacco smoke exposure and ischaemic heart disease: an evaluation of evidence. *BMJ.* 1997; 315: 973 – 80.

[14] Leone A. *Statistics findings by questionnaires: problems with answers on smoking.* Conference (unpublished) at the International Meeting on Smoking and Health, Lerici, Italy, May 1996.

[15] Leone A. Passive smoking causes cardiac alterations in post-MI subjects. *Int. J. Smoking Cessation.* 1996; 3: 42 – 3.

Chapter 8

EPIDEMIOLOGICAL STUDIES

ABSTRACT

A large series of clinico-epidemiological studies, particularly cohort studies and case-control studies, and metanalyses would seem to conclude that there is a negative relationship between passive smoking exposure and cardiovascular system, although the reached results are not unanimous for all types of findings.

In family homes as well as in workplaces, environmental tobacco smoke exposure is associated with an increased risk of coronary heart disease in exposed nonsmokers when they are compared to unexposed nonsmokers. Both fatal and nonfatal coronary events have been seen.

A significantly negative effect on carotid artery wall induced by passive smoking has been well identified by the largest observational study conducted. Carotid artery intimal-medial thickness increased significantly after exposure to passive smoking in never smokers. In contrast, further studies conducted by different statistical methodologies and metanalyses on the relationship between passive smoking exposure and cerebrovascular disease and stroke would be needed in an attempt to establish whether there really exists an association between the two manifestations. However, there are always more up-to-data observations that seem to show an increased risk in cerebrovascular disease and stroke after exposure to passive smoking.

Keywords: Passive smoking, cohort study, case-control study, coronary heart disease, arterial wall, cerebrovascular disease, stroke.

Nowadays, there is no doubt that exposure to passive smoking leads to only one result ,which is a reversibly functional harm of the heart and blood vessels following acute exposure, and pathologic alterations that become, in the long run, irreversible lesions of the above target organs after chronic exposure [1–7]. Therefore, the American Heart Association has included passive smoking among the major risk factors for heart disease in both adults and children [6].

No country is free from this problem, which plagues developing and developed countries alike, although with different results due to different lifestyles, smoking habits, educational and socio-economic conditions, diffusion of antismoking campaigns. The different continents and countries registered (Table 8.1.) in the past (eighth decade) smoking rates per year, in both male and female adults, are different from each other [8].

Table 8.1. Smoking rates for adults in different continents and countries

Country/Continent	Male (percent)	Female (percent)	Year
America	37	28	1980
Australia	38	33	1979
Asia	44	14	1990
Europe	34	32	1983
Sweden	31	30	1982
Japan	73	15	1979

Morever, analyzing separately the different countries of each continent, there is evidence of a different distribution of yearly cigarette consumption country by country that is unrelated to the degree of developing.

This can clearly be seen by the analysis of cigarette consumption in Asia [9], where there are countries [10] with a high level of industrial and technologic development, countries developing quickly, and countries poorly developed. Figure 8.1. shows yearly cigarette consumption in this geographic area. Observed consumption would seem to depend not only by the degree of developing, but mainly by different lifestyles, locally inveterate habits and socio-economic conditions.

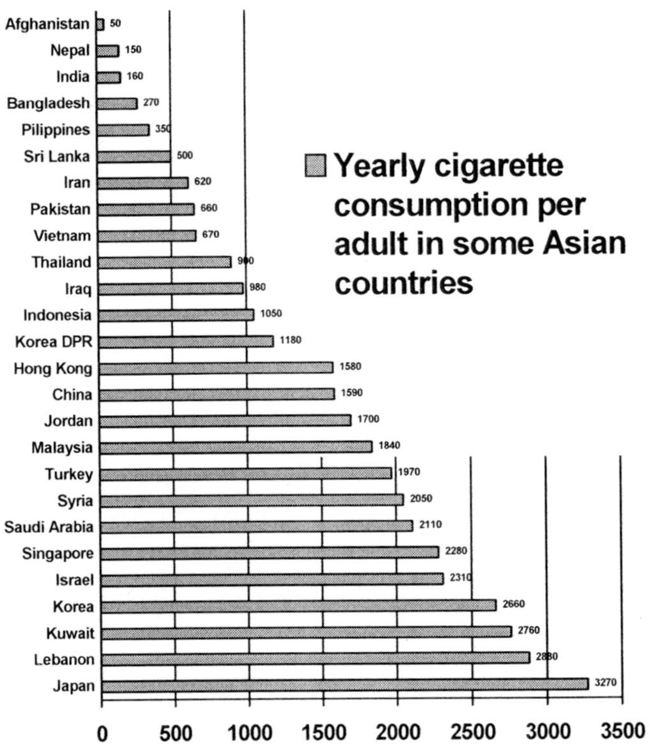

Figure 8.1. Yearly cigarette consumption in different countries of Asia. It may be seen a wide different habit smoking for country by country (years 1985 – 88, mean).

It may be seen that, in percentage, developed countries like Japan, Israel, Singapore, and others (Figure 8.2.) have a mean yearly consumption of smoked cigarette equal to 52%, quickly developing countries equal to 29%, and poorly developed countries equal to 19%. Asia Continent would seem to have, epidemiologically, a different smoking habit than that showed by different continent countries like Europe and North America where developed countries register a reduction in yearly cigarette consumption. Since exposure to passive smoking is a direct consequence of both number of active smokers and number of smoked cigarettes, it can be deduced that passive smoking in "smoking" countries can cause more evident damage to exposed people.

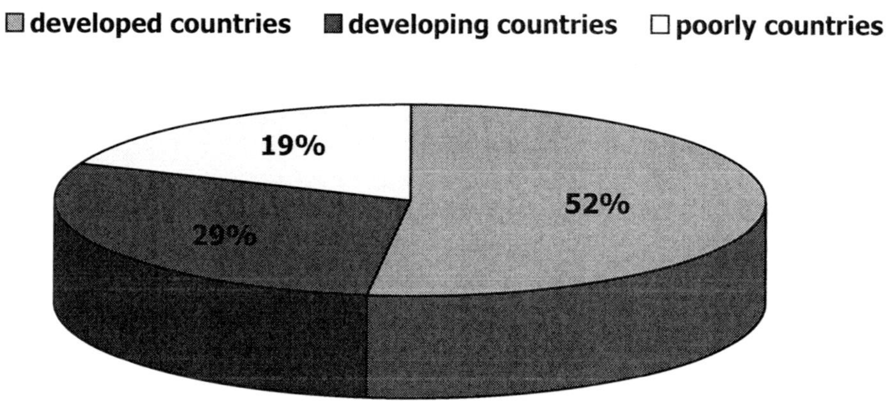

Figure 8.2. Smoking distribution (percent) between developed, developing and poorly developed countries.

About the type of studies, all types of epidemiological studies on the effect of passive smoking exposure on cardiovascular system have been conducted: observational and experimental studies.

Among observational studies, mainly cohort-studies and case-control studies have been analyzed. The whole studies, however, came from different countries with different populations examined. Therefore, studies by metanalysis were also evaluated for better assessing the degree of damage.

Findings have been conducted particularly on the relationship between passive smoking exposure and coronary heart disease, although vascular alterations due to passive smoking have been examined more and more by several researchers. Thus, vascular pathology seems to be a close manifestation of secondhand smoke.

Observational Studies

Observational findings on the relationship between passive smoking and cardiovascular alterations have begun to be conducted since the eighth decade, having death from ischemic heart disease as the main end-point. Later, several different end-points have been evaluated and data about anatomical changes of heart and vessel structures were also analyzed as well as metabolic alterations, particularly concerning lipid profile. However, the majority of the reports concerned fatal coronary events in non-smoking women exposed at home to smoke from their husbands' cigarettes. Cohort-studies, case-control studies and studies conducted by metanalysis provide effective results nowadays to establish the cardiovascular damage from passive smoking.

North America, Asia, and some north countries of Europe have primarily conducted this type of findings. Later, studies became widespread, although such an occurence enlarged study population on one hand while on the other hand, it contributed to increased confusion on the amount of cardiovascular damage. Parameters such as race, age, gender, social class, clinical and metabolic values, that were different in measurement level with regard to the standard values of different laboratoires, were shared without any statistical reason. Yet several papers mixed all these data in an attempt to demonstrate the significant existence of an undoubted damage deriving from passive smoking. By doing so, they involuntarily supported the opinions, based primarily on the inadequate use of really appropriate statistical methods, capable of demonstrate the damage of all those persons who defined worthless or almost absent cardiovascular alterations from passive smoking. Indeed, damage exists to the strongest level and it may be easily demonstrated by a correct analysis, conducted without prejudice, of the results that several studies provide.

Cohort-Studies

Cohort studies of secondhand smoke exposure concerning primarily the risk of development or clinical and pathologic impairment of a pre-existing coronary heart disease are listed in Table 8.2.

Table 8.2. Main cohort studies of passive smoking exposure in never smokers

Population study (number, gender, exposure)	Reference (Author, number)	Follow-up (years)	End-points (main)
91,540 women (husbands' smoke)	Hirayama (11)	16	death from CHD
695 women (husbands' smoke)	Garland et al. (12)	10	death from CHD
1,245 men (wives' smoke)	Svendsen et al.(13)	7	death from CHD
6,507 women (husbands' smoke)	Butler (14)	6	death fromCHD
12,348 women+3,488 men(mixed)	Helsing et al. (15)	12	death from CHD
1,784 women+671 men (mixed)	Hole et al. (16)	11.5	death from CHD
14,873 women+4,162 men (home)	Sandler et al. (17)	12	death from CHD
513 women (husbands' smoke)	Humble et al. (18)	20	death from CHD
247,412 women+88,458 men(spouse)	LeVois et al. (19)	13	death from CHD
353,180 women+126,500 men (all)	Steenland et al.(20)	8	death from CHD
32,046 women (home, workplace)	Kawachi et al. (21)	10	myocardial infarction, and death from CHD

Abbreviations: mixed= cohabitant smoked; spouse= spouse smoked; all= smoke everywhere; CHD= coronary heart disease.

From the analysis of Table 8.2, one can see that among the enrolled populations, female gender is widely numerically prevailing, although the number of men included in several studies is statistically valid for a correct estimate. No data about children exposure are provided by these studies. Totally, studied population consisted of 985,422 subjects, whose 760,898 (77%) were women and 224,524 men (23%). Although statistically, the number of studied population, permits effective estimates, there are some limits in expressing an objective estimate due to the different types and sites of the exposure and follow-up duration – it is known that structural alterations of the cardiovascular system develop over a long time. Therefore, it is easier is to find anatomical alterations - generic end-point established, death from coronary heart disease, when the follow-up period is longer. Alternate apprasels are presented by Kawachi and al., where myocardial infarction is analyzed as the first end-point, and other studies which propose major coronary risk factors.

Reached conclusions in all these studies cannot be attributed to an equal parameter of statistical estimate. This statement is supported by the analysis of the relative risk, namely the risk by which people have the possibility to be damaged with a major frequency when they are compared to people having no risk. It varies, sometimes widely, in the different findings (Table 8.3.) with no association with a follow-up study.

Table 8.3. Relative risk (95% confidence interval) and follow-up duration

Author	Reference	Follow-up duration (years)	Relative risk
LeVois/Layard	19	13	1 (0.97 – 1.04)
Hirayama	11	16	1.18 (0.98 – 1.41)
Steenland et al.	20	8	1.23 (1.03 – 1.47)
Sandler et al.	17	12	1.22 (1.09 – 1.37)
Helsing et al.	15	12	1.27 (1.10 – 1.60)
Butler	14	6	1.40 (0.51 – 3.84)
Humble et al.	18	20	1.59 (0.99 – 2.57)
Kawachi et al.	21	10	1.71 (1.03 – 2.84)
Hole et al.	16	11.5	2.01 (1.21 – 3.35)
Svendsen et al.	13	7	2.23 (0.72 – 6.92)
Garland et al.	12	10	2.70 (0.59 – 12.33)

Moreover, the relative risk is not increasing with the increase of the number of subjects enrolled in the different studies. However, as mentioned before, such a fact could be due to epidemiolojical differences in the studied population.

Thus, it would be better to analyze the cohort-studies separately rather than after their grouping in an attempt to find the real level of damage caused by passive smoking exposure on cardiovascular system.

In Hirayama study, among 91,540 nonsomker women exposed to passive smoking, 494 died from coronary heart disease. Compared to nonsmoking women married to nonsmokers, the relative risk of women married to ex-smokers or heavy smokers, varied from respectively 1.10 and 1.31. When the analysis was adjusted according to the age of husbands as well as their working, one could observe an increase in relative risk of passively exposed women.

The difference interval in the relative risk of this finding was too small to permit certain conclusions, although there was evidence of a major risk in passive smoking exposed women.

Garland and coworkers analyzed a small number of exposed women (695 subjects). After 10 year follow-up there were 19 women who died from coronary heart disease . The relative risk was statistically significant since it was estimated that the possibility that exposed women underwent fatal outcome with a frequency of about three times more that that of non-exposed women. A limit to these observations could be the small number of enrolled subjects that is however statistically sufficient to permit a significant estimate. Moreover, the duration of follow-up (10 years) strengthens the possibility of the cardiovascular damage from passive smoking in exposed never smokers.

Svendsen and coworkers' paper reached the conclusion that the risk in developing cardiovascular events affected both never smoker men and men who were nonsmokers exposed to wives' smoking at the enrollment in the study. The relative risk for this study reached an estimate of 2.23 during a follow-up of 7 years. Moreover, the number of enrolled subjects was of 1,245 people and therefore, there were presuppositions of a statistical analysis people had also been included in the Multiple Risk Factor Intervention Trial (MRFIT), a study that, as we will see later, could reach very interesting conclusions on the role of several major coronary risk factors. A limitation of this study was that the study population belonged to only 18 United States cities and therefore, it was not representative of the entire population as well as enrolled men, who were at a high risk of cardiovascular event since their serum cholesterol concentrations, as well as diastolic blood pressure, reached elevated measures.

Butler's cohort study had a follow-up duration of 6 years, analyzed a large sample of women (6,507), who were exposed to their husbands' smoke, and relative risk reached an estimate of 1.40. Risk was calculated also in some men who were not current smokers and exposure to smoke in the home and workplace was also considered. The conclusions of the follow-up suggested that the exposure to environmental tobacco smoke at home and at work increased the risk of heart disease mortality in nonsmoking women but not in never smoking men. Moreover, passive smoking exposure from work was of border-line statistical significance. No evident reason could explain the difference in results by gender in this finding. On the contrary, the higher risk in home exposure could be reasonably attributed to the longer time of in-house living.

The role of environmental tobacco smoke exposure in the etiology of heart disease, fatal events in both women and men, was investigated by Helsing and coworkers. In the never smokers, there were a total of 370 deaths in men and 988 in women for whom coronary heart disease was listed as the underlying cause of death. Positive characteristics in this study was particularly the large sample of analyzed subjects either of female gender or male gender. Moreover, relative risk denoted that there was a mortality rate from cardiovascular events that was about one and a half times more elevated for the exposed never smokers, and the studied sample had almost similar habits since it came from a well bordered geographic area (West Maryland).

The Scottish study conducted by Hole and coworkers recorded a relative risk of possible cardiovascular events equal to 2.01 for the exposed subjects who were women with a number of two and a half times greater than that of men. The study sample was significant for a correct statistical approach, and a follow-up duration of 11.5 years permitted a careful estimate of reached results. Two end-points characterized this study: investigating the risk of cardiorespiratory symptoms and assessing the mortality from coronary heart disease in a well bordered geographic area like western Scotland. The effects of passive smoking did not impair in a statistically significant way clinical symptoms and electrocardiographic patterns of coronary heart disease in exposed nonsmokers when they were compared to the control group. The effects of passive smoking exposure were more evident for fatal coronary heart disease events. Passive smokers experienced a higher age and gender-adjusted mortality rate of coronary heart disease than controls. Exposed never smokers died about two times more frequently than those from the control group. A great advantage in this finding is that the whole study sample came from a bordered county of only two towns. Moreover, a careful adjustment in the analysis of some other risk factors like age, gender, social class, diastolic blood pressure and serum cholesterol concentration made obtained results worthwhile to be estimated by a statistically correct approach.

The findings of Sandler and coworkers concerned the largest statistical sample with similar racial characteristics (white race). Women exceeded men numerically by a large amount – respectively 14,873 vs 4,162 - and exposure to passive smoking occurred in home from any household member who smoked. Results related to death from coronary heart disease of nonsmokers exposed to secondhand smoke were supported by a relative risk of 1.22 for 12 years of follow-up. Findings were conducted in residents of Maryland. Controlled variables in this study were age, marital status, years of schooling, and quality of housing. The latter is a social factor of remarkable importance, considered only in a few studies like Helsing and coworkers study, to carefully evaluate the type of exposure in view of the role that environment plays in inducing cardiovascular damage (see also Chapter 1, section 1.5). Observations in this study recorded a risk of death from coronary heart disease that is close to other findings, although with a lower level when it is compared with relative risk found by Kawachi, Hole, Svendsen and Garland.

The association between passive smoking exposure and mortality rate from coronary heart disease was investigated among nonsmoking women in Evans County, Georgia, by Humble and coworkers. Results on environmental tobacco exposure were presented for all subjects combined, and separately by race and social class. Occupation, education, income of the head of each family as studied parameters were also considered. A relative risk of 1.59 for 20 year follow-up duration affected study sample that was numerically small (513 women exposed to husbands' smoke). All mortality due to cardiovascular disease (including also strokes) listed as an underlying cause of death derived from death certificates which were also considered in result analysis. Age, serum cholesterol level, diastolic blood pressure and body mass index were controlled variables. Nonsmoking women married to current smokers had a higher risk for coronary heart disease mortality than women married to never smokers. Increased risk was observed particularly for all black women and white women of higher social status but not for white women of low social class. The findings do not provide explanations for this inconsistent data. Moreover, the small number of enrolled subjects, together with the division of the results to different subgroups, make this finding hard to be statistically estimated.

The largest studies of passive smoking exposure and coronary heart disease are based on two American Cancer Society cohort studies: Cancer Prevention Study 1 (CPS 1) and Cancer Prevention Study II (CPS –II). LeVois and Layard analyzed the CPS-I data and found no relationship between smoking by a spouse and coronary heart disease. Data from CPS-II were analyzed independently by LeVois and Layard and by Steenland and coworkers. These two reports based on essentially the same data reached different findings, probably because they used different definitions of exposure to environmental tobacco smoke. LeVois and Layard defined exposure as marriage to someone who was a past or current smoker. By doing so, they found no association between coronary heart disease and smoking exposure. On the contrary, Steenland and coworkers separated out current and past smokers, on the grounds that current environmental tobacco smoke exposure would be expected to have a greater impact on coronary heart disease risk than past environmental tobacco smoke exposure. Furthermore, in a subgroup analysis, subjects were included only when their responses about the smoking status of the spouse were in agreement with self-report from that spouse. In this analysis, never smoker men married to women who were smokers at the entry to the study had a relative risk of fatal heart disease of 1.23 (95% confidence interval: 1.03 – 1.47), and never smoker women married to smoking men had a relative risk of 1.19 (95% confidence interval: 0.97 – 1.45).

Finally, the findings of Kawachi and coworkers examined the largest sample of 32,046 nonsmoker women, exposed to passive smoking everywhere, particularly in the home and workplace, for a follow-up duration of 10 years. They had a mean relative risk of 1.71, totally considered for all types of exposure. When authors examined a subgroup of women who were not exposed to environmental tobacco smoke at home but at work, interesting observations emerged. Among these women, there was some evidence that regular exposure to environmental tobacco smoke at work increased the risk of coronary heart disease with a relative risk estimate of 1.92 (95% confidence interval: 0.88 – 4.18).

From the analysis of the above cohort studies, there is evidence that conflicting results may be provided about the degree of risk for the development of coronary and generally cardiovascular disease following exposure to passive smoking. Of significant importance to support this statement are the two papers of LeVois/Layard and Steenland and coworkers who reached different results analyzing the same data, but using a different statistical approach. Moreover, all findings are based on a confidence interval of statistical significance of 95%. Nevertheless, estimating the mean of relative risk of all above cohort studies, we find a value of 1.75 that is representative of the fact that just less than two individuals exposed to passive smoking can undergo both nonfatal or fatal cardiovascular event when compared to individuals never exposed. Thus, as one can see, braving the danger from passive smoking is an occurence to avoid carefully as the above reports show, although some important limits, seem to show.

Case-Control Studies

In contrast to the cohort studies, which provide results not always related to the demonstration of an evident damage of the heart and blood vessels due to passive smoking exposure, case-control studies may follow different ways. In each study, the history of passive smoking by the patient was obtained by an interview from lifelong non-smoking patients with coronary heart disease or where the illness was rapidly fatal, by interview or questionnaire involving the next of kin or a close relative. Collected data were compared with equivalent data from non-smoking individuals without symptomatic coronary heart disease. Although it is generally held that the control groups drawn from the general population are to be preferred to comparisons made with patients admitted to hospital with diseases other than coronary heart disease, all studies did not satisfy this standard. Moreover, there are also some variations among different investigations with regard to the definition of a case of coronary heart disease, and the sources of passive exposure to tobacco smoke. Some studies included only men, others only women, and some both sexes [22 – 25]. Yet, several data collected by answers to questionnaires could show some of those limits explained in the previous chapter.

It is basic, in my opinion, to confirm again that the large number of subjects enrolled in each of these studies, rather than a compared investigation of every parameter under study in the different papers, validate statistically the results obtained. Such a fact is further demonstrated by the different end-points which characterize some investigations with regard to others as well as by the lack of similar variables which to be analyzed in different findings, notwithstanding some of these variables were often related to other major coronary risk factors and therefore, capable to influence the final result of the observed responses. However, statistically adjusted parameters for some variables calculated in several reports could limit the effects of the above statements.

Table 8.4. lists the main case-control studies conducted by different researchers to assess cardiovascular damage due to passive smoking.

Table 8.4. Case-control studies of passive smoking and risk of CHD among never smokers

Population study (number, gender, exposure)	Controls	Reference (Author, number)	RR (95% CI)
41 men,77 women, spouse (CHD)	133 men, 318 women (hospital admitted)	Lee et al.(26)	1.03 (0.65 – 1.62)
34 women husband (hospital pts)	68 women (34 hospital pts, 34 non)	He et al. (27)	1.5 (1.3 –1.8)
44 men,22women,home/work (MI or death from CHD)	84 men,174 women (MI or death from CHD)	Jackson (28)	1.85 (0.3-12.6) 3.45 (0.2 – 35.2)
183men,160women,home/work (MI or death from CHD)	293 men,174 women (hospital pts)	Dobson et al.(23)	1.75 (0.5-4.1)
69 men,44 women , spouse (acute MI)	161 men,56 women (hospital pts)	La Vecchia et al.(29)	1.21 (0.57-2.52)
59 women, husband/work (CHD)	126 pts (hospital pts)	He et al. (25)	2.36 (1.01-5.55)
475 men,914 women, spouse (death from heart disease)	998 men,1,930 women (death from other cause)	Layard (30)	1.0 (0.7-1.3)
68 men,46 women,home/work (MI, hospital)	108 men,50 women (hospital,no CHD)	Muscat/Wynder(24)	2.4 (1.1 – 4.8)
70 men and women, any exp (CHD)	2,278 men – women (CHD)	Tunstall-Pedoe et al.(31)	1.5 (0.9-2.6)
336 men and women,spouse (acute MI, hospital)	446 pts (hospital pts)	Ciruzzi et al. (32)	1.68 (1.2-2.37)
686men,267women,home/work (fatal,non fatal MI)	3,189 residents (same communities)	McElduff et al.(33)	1.41 (0.73-2.71)
All nonfatal MIs, spouse (199 men, 135 women)	401 men,276 women (hospital crowding area)	Rosenlund et al.(34)	1.37 (0.9-2.09)

Abbreviations: RR= relative risk; CI= confidence interval; CHD= coronary heart disease; pts= patients; MI= myocardial infarction.

Since the role of the analysis of variables to be examined related to different studies has been suggested, it is important to know which of these variables were considered.

Several variables were analyzed in the above case-control studies. Some of these were related to biologic characteristics of the enrolled subjects, some to lifestyle, and some more to geographical areas where case-control study was conducted. Major coronary risk factors could also affect studied population. Moreover, as case-control findings demand, there were study subjects followed as cases and subjects as a control group who was not affected by the examined disease. Table 8.5. lists the main controlled variables assessed in the different control-case studies.

Table 8.5. Variables controlled in examined case-control studies

Author's Reference (reference number)	Controlled variables
26	Age, gender, hospital region.
27	Alcohol consumption, exercise,personal and family history of CHD, hypertension, lipid profile
29	Age, social status, history of CHD.
23	Age, history of MI.
29	Age, gender, body mass index, coffee consumption, social status, lipid profile, hypertension, diabetes mellitus, family history of MI.
25	Age, hypertension, personality type, lipids.
30	Age, race.
24	Age, housing, lipid profile, diastolic blood pressure.
31	Age, gender, race, education, hypertension.
32	Age, gender, race, education, body mass index, lipid profile, diabetes mellitus, CHD, hypertension.
33	Age, education, history of CHD, body mass index.
34	Age, gender, hospital area, body mass index, social status, job, hypertension, diet, diabetes mellitus.

From the analysis of the controlled variables listed in Table 8.5, there is evidence that in several studies, large but very different statistical combinations have been associated with the results deriving from passive smoking exposure, as in the cohort studies. Moreover, some of these controlled variables acted as major cardiovascular risk factors. In view of the possibility of confounding estimates when the case-control studies are analyzed statistically together, it could be a good procedure to follow the methodologic approach of the researcher who planned the study and then, separately estimate the reached results, with each finding different from one another. However, this approach could not provide equal observations in the different studies because of an unsimilar level of risk and obtained results. Therefore, some remarks on the role of the above case-control studies need to be discussed.

In the analysis concerned with exposure of never smoking women to their husbands' tobacco smoke, three out of five studies experienced that passive smoking was a factor that increased the risk of coronary heart disease. Moreover, two of the studies were statistically significant at a 5% level. Only three studies clarified the results of men exposure to their wives' smoke. One of these suggested that there was an increase in cardiovascular risk, while the others showed a small decrease, and none were statistically significant.

Three case-control studies analyzed the exposure to environmental tobacco smoke in the workplace and the risk of coronary heart disease. Among women, the study of Dobson and coworkers found a non-significant reduction in risk, Muscat and Wynder found no effect at all, and the study by He and coworkers appeared in the British Medical Journal 1994, reporting a non-significant increase.

The first published study to investigate the effects of passive smoking at work on the risk of coronary heart disease in men was conducted by Dobson and coworkers in Australia. This study found no association. More recently, Muscat and Wynder reported an odd ratio, namely the ratio of the probability of an event occurring to that of its not occurring, of 1.2 (95% confidence interval: 0.6 – 2.2) for exposure of men to environmental tobacco smoke at work.

The case-control study of Layard is almost double the size of the six other case-control studies. The study compared spouse smoking between cases who died from coronary heart disease and controls who died from other diseases, excluding those people who died from diseases that are known to be strongly related to smoking. The use of dead controls is problematic as factors causing premature death (such as smoking) tend to be over-represented among those who have died. Passive smoking exposure could be more common among dead controls than among living controls, resulting in underestimation of the strength of association between passive smoking and coronary heart disease.

Two excellent reports [35 – 36] on the epidemiologic significance of cardiovascular damage from passive smoking exposure in case-control studies explain in detail the statistical parameter estimate, type of studied population, geographic and socio-economic characteristics, controlled variables analyzed, and so on. Thus, by these reports, one can have much more information about the epidemiological characteristics of the subjects included in case-control studies. Such a subject does not belong to the purposes of this chapter that sets to discuss the role of case-control studies in an overall way, in an attempt to clarify the obtained results in people exposed to passive smoking.

However, these two excellent reports did not mention the findings conducted on nonsmoker women in the geographic area of Xi'an, China, by He and coworkers [37]. In my opinion, these findings are worthwhile to mention.

In this study, the coronary heart disease cases included some women in whom the diagnosis was based on the demonstration of coronary artery narrowings by coronary angiography. Moreover, He and coworkers extended this work by conducting a cross-sectional study (namely a type of study where a statistical analysis of variations in data obtained from a set of sources at the same time is estimated) of 161 women who had coronary angiography because of suspected coronary heart disease. This investigation found that higher levels of exposure to passive smoking at home were associated with a greater number of atherosclerotic coronary arteries with a highly statistical significance (p less than 0.01).

This case-control study is to be considered one of the most significant to demonstrate structural lesions of the coronary tree after prolonged exposure to passive smoking.

However, none of the cohort or case-control studies to date has validated the history of active or passive smoking by measuring constituents of smoke or their metabolites in the body fluid or exhaled air of the enrolled subjects. The level of cotinine, the main metabolite of nicotine, was measured in the blood of participants in a cross-sectional study in Scotland, that included primarily cases of angina and diagnosed coronary heart disease plus additional cases of "undiagnosed" coronary heart disease defined by typical electrocardiographic changes [38]. In this survey, the prevalence of angina, that was defined by responses to a standardised questionnaire and a previous diagnosis of coronary heart disease among biochemically-confirmed nonsmokers, more than doubled across categories of response to a question about exposure to passive smoke. This trend was not as marked for undiagnosed coronary heart disease. Moreover, when the nonsmokers were subdivided into four subgroups on the basis of their serum cotinine, only the prevalence of diagnosed coronary heart disease was significantly greater in those with the highest levels of the metabolite. These conclusions would suggest that there was a clear relationship between cotinine levels and ischemic heart disease, and serum cotinine levels derived from passive smoking exposure.

In conclusion, case-control studies have produced inconsistent findings on the relationship between passive smoking exposure and coronary heart disease. In contrast, most cohort studies, although with the described limits of statistical estimate for some of these, have identified an increased risk of coronary heart disease following passive smoking exposure.

Metanalysis Studies

The metanalyses of studies on the relationship between passive smoking exposure and coronary heart disease have been conducted by different researchers in an attempt to establish further the "real" role of the exposure to passive smoking. Exposure to passive smoking may be influenced by a large series of factors that might differ in studies conducted separately.

The main metanalyses of passive smoking exposure and risk of coronary heart disease are listed in Table 8.6.

Among the different metanalysis studies, the study of Wells [4] is worthwhile to be discussed. Wells conducted a metanalysis of 12 epidemiological studies of smoking by a spouse and the risk of coronary heart disease. Seven studies were cohort studies having nonfatal coronary events as outcome, and 5 case-control studies analyzed fatal coronary events. He estimated that passive smoking was associated with a 23 % increase in risk of death from coronary heart disease in women, and a 25 % of increased risk in men. For nonfatal coronary events, the author found a 51 % increase in risk in women and a 28 % increase in risk for men.

Law and Hackshaw [42] also conducted a metanalysis of 12 studies to establish a possible relationship between passive smoking and coronary heart disease. Authors calculated a pooled relative risk of 1.3 (95% confidence interval from 1.2 to 1.4). However, this metanalysis did not analyze results for men and women separately.

Both the metanalyses included 12 studies with 10 studies in common. Differently, two studies in metanalyses included two observational studies for the metanalysis of Wells, and two papers that had been published after Wells had completed his work for the metanalysis of Law and Hackshaw.

From the epidemiology of observational studies, one can observe [4] that an increase of coronary heart disease risk varying from 20% to 70% characterized those subjects who had had passive smoking exposure from spousal or household environmental tobacco smoke and that an increase in risk is not explained by misclassification of smokers as nonsmokers or by association with the other major coronary risk factors. However, whatever the limit might be, the large majority of the observational studies on the relationship between passive smoking exposure and risk of ischemic heart disease demonstrates an increased risk of coronary events in exposed people.

Table 8.6. Main metanalyses of passive smoking exposure and coronary heart disease

Study design		Reference	Outcome	Combined RR(men,women) (95% confidence interval)
Cohort studies	(7:Garland et al. 1985, Svendsen et al. 1987, Butler 1988, Hole et al. 1989,Sandler et al. 1989, Hirayama 1990, Humble et al. 1990)	Wells (4)	Non fatal coronary events	1.42 (1.15 – 1.75)
Case-control studies	(5 : Lee et al.1986, He 1989, Jackson 1989, Dobson et al. 1991, He et al. 1994)		Fatal coronary events	1.23 (1.12 – 1.38)
Cohort studies	(9 : Garland et al. 1985, Svendsen et al. 1987, Butler 1988, Hole et al. 1989,Sandler et al. 1989, Hirayama 1990, Humble et al. 1990, Steenland et al. 1996, Kawachi et al. 1997)	Law et al.(39)	All coronary events	1.30 (1.22 – 1.38)
Case-control	(10 : Lee et al.1986, He 1989, Jackson 1989 Dobson et al. 1991, Lee 1992,La Vecchia, et al. 1993, He et al. 1994, Muscat/Wynder 1995, Tunstall-Pedoe et al.1995, Ciruzzi et al. 1998)			1.30 (1.22 – 1.38)
Cohort studies	(10 : Hirayama 1984, Garland et al 1985, Svendsen et al. 1987, Butler 1988, Hole et al. 1989, Sandler et al. 1989, Hirayama 1990, Humble et al. 1990, Steenland et al. 1996, Kawachi et al. 1997)	He et al.(40)	All coronary events	1.25 (1.17 – 1.32)
Case-control studies	(8 : Lee et al. 1986, He1989, Jackson 1989, Dobson et al. 1991, La Vecchia et al. 1993, He et al. 1994, Muscat/Wynder 1995, Ciruzzi et al. 1998)			1.51 (1.26 – 1.81)
Cohort studies	(10 :Hirayama 1984, Garland et al. 1985, Svendsen et al. 1987,Butler1988, Hole et al. 1989, Sandler et al. 989,Hirayama1990, Humble et al. 1990, LeVois/Layard1995, Steenland et al. 1996)	Thun et al.(41)	All coronary events	1.25 (1.17 – 1.33)
Case-control	(8 : Lee et al.1986, He1989, Jackson 1989, Dobson et al. 1991, La Vecchia et al. 1993, He et al.1994, Muscat/Wynder1995,		Nonfatal coronary events	1.32 (1.04 – 1.67)
	Ciruzzi et al.1998)		Fatal coronary events	1.22 (1.14 – 1.30)

Epidemiology of Vascular Studies: The Arterial Wall

As aforesaid, cigarette smoking has been shown to be one of the strongest predictors of atherosclerotic plaque progression [43].

Notwithstanding such a statement was known for many years, observational studies on the relationship between passive smoking and peripheral artery disease have begun to appear later than those concerning coronary artery disease. That occurred in spite of the high incidence of cerebrovascular diseases, primarily strokes, in smokers [17, 26, 44 – 48]. Six studies (Table 8.7.) have examined the association between passive smoking and risk of stroke. Four studies were case-control studies, one cohort study and one cross-sectional study. They analyzed passive smoking exposure in home and workplace, and one very recent study [48] assessed smoking and cotinine measurement.

To find metabolites of passive smoking components in biologic fluids, particularly urine, of never smokers, is the most significant factor capable of demonstrating that exposure to passive smoking has surely occurred and then the dosage of cotinine should be conducted, at least in small- scale studies, when results to attribute to passive smoking must be fully evaluated. In my opinion, this is the reason to emphasize the results of the paper conducted by Whincup and coworkers.

Table 8.7. Passive smoking exposure and cerebrovascular disease and stroke in different epidemiological studies

Type of study	Conclusions
Case-control study (Lee et al., 1986)	No association between spousal passive smoke and stroke.
Case-control study (Donnan et al.1989)	No association between parental passive smoke and stroke.
Cohort study (Sandler et al. 1989)	No association between home passive smoking and stroke.
Cross-sectional study(Howard et al.1998)	No association between all source passive smoke and cerebrovascular disease.
Case-control study (Bonita et al. 1999)	Association between home passive smoking and acute stroke in both sexes.
Case-control study (You et al. 1999)	No association between spousal passive smoke and stroke.

As one can see, a strong association between passive smoking exposure and cerebrovascular disease, primarily stroke, was clearly not found in all studies unless for the study of Bonita and coworkers. In my opinion, the latter study is an excellent study that carefully analyzes important variables related to cardiovascular risk and follows the diagnostic criteria of stroke defined by the World Health Organization.

A significant breakthrough in the study of vascular disease, primarily atherosclerosis, has been the use of B-mode ultrasound for measuring arterial intimal-medial thickness as a surrogate end-point for the degree of atherosclerosis and its progression.

One of the largest studies followed carotid artery intimal-medial thickness over a three year duration in black and white men and women, aged from 45 to 65 years, enrolled for the Atherosclerosis Risk in Communities Study (ARIC) [49]. 10,914 participants were enrolled in the study from 1987 to 1989. 4,298 people had had exposure to environmental tobacco smoke, some had been past smokers and some never smokers. Compared to nonsmokers who had had no exposure anyway to smoke, active smokers showed a 50% increase in carotid artery intimal-medial thickness, but also nonsmokers exposed had an increase in this parameter of 20%. Dividing study population into five subgroups, nonsmokers with no passive smoking exposure, nonsmokers with passive smoking exposure, past smokers with no passive smoking exposure, past smokers with passive smoking exposure, and current smokers, interesting observations (Table 8.8.) emerge from this finding.

Table 8.8. Total study population and carotid artery intimal-medial thickening

Subject characteristic	Smoking Exposure (yes, no)	Number	IMT thickness (μm)
Nonsmokers	no	2316	26.9
Nonsmokers	yes	2449	32.7
Past smokers	no	1344	33.4
Past smokers	yes	1849	39.8
Active smokers	yes	2956	41.2

Abbreviation: IMT= intimal-medial thickness.

Non exposed never smokers had a lower intimal-medial thickness of the carotid artery when they were compared to those people who had had smoking exposure either active exposure or passive exposure. Moreover, current smokers showed a maximum amount in wall thickness. Therefore, exposure to passive smoking identified a significant amount in the arterial wall thickness.

A critical question could be whether these ultrasound recorded intimal- medial thickness changes are valid surrogate markers for the progression of atherosclerosis [50]. There is evidence that carotid artery intimal-medial thickness would be well related to the prevalence of atherosclerotic lesions in other arteries. Indeed, two recent studies [51–52] identify a relationship between increased intimal-medial thickness and progression in cardiovascular disease. In over 1,000 Finnish men, Salonen and Salonen [51] observed that each millimetre increase in carotid artery intimal-medial thickness increased the risk of an acute coronary event of 2.14 fold. Similar results were observed by Bots and coworkers [52].

One can therefore deduce that changes in carotid artery intimal-medial thickness caused by environmental tobacco smoke exposure identify a progression of arterial wall changes that lead to atherosclerosis. Coronary arteries may also be included in these mechanisms.

In conclusion, although observational studies do not permit to reach the certainty about a negative relationship between passive smoking exposure and cerebrovascular disease or acute stroke, these studies are numerically small. Some of these studies, however, provide information that a relationship exists. Moreover, evaluating the course of arterial thickness after exposure to passive smoking, and the study that identifies a significant damage from passive smoking exposure is the largest numerically on the subject, and there is clear evidence of vascular damage from environmental tobacco smoke. Therefore, statistical methodologies, applied in different epidemiological studies should be re-examined and studies by metanalysis, notwithstanding their limits.

The epidemiological data collected by the analysis of the results in observational studies support a negative relationship between passive smoking exposure and cardiovascular disease, although with some specific characteristics, particularly when spouses are responsible of the event. Some types of disease are of primarily interest: ischemic heart disease for what concerns the heart, and carotid intimal-medial thickness for what is concerning vascular tree. Studies on cerebrovascular disease and stroke are yet to be developed to assess whether passive smoking exposure negatively influence the phenomenon. Probably, the changes in lipid profile, that assumes an atherogenic pattern with a decrease in HDL-Cholesterol and an increase in LDL-Cholesterol after exposure to passive smoking, explain carotid alterations more than cerebrovascular changes. It is known that carotid artery is a blood vessel where lipid deposits may cause atherosclerotic plaques with a markedly major incidence than in other arterial tree locations, and these changes are comparable to what coronary arteries can similarly show. On the contrary, cerebral arteries feel less than these phenomena particularly because of their anatomic characteristics.

These observations, demonstrate that cardiovascular system is clinically a target organ for passive smoking, and also for those reports that do not identify a statistically significant increase in cardiovascular events after exposure to passive smoking, however, have shown, sometimes, events of the same degree or reduced incidence when they were compared to observations of non exposed subjects. In all cases, passive smoking exposure increased cardiovascular risk.

References

[1] Leone A, Mori L, Bertanelli F, Fabiano P, Filippelli M. Indoor passive smoking: its effects on cardiac performance. *Int. J. Cardiol.* 1991; 8: 247 – 52.

[2] Glantz SA, Parmley WW. Passive smoking and heart disease : epidemiology, physiology, and biochemistry. *Circulation.* 1991; 83: 1 – 12.

[3] Leone A. The heart: a target organ for cigarette smoking. *J. Smoking-Related Dis.* 1992; 3: 197 –201.

[4] Wells AG. Passive smoking as a cause of heart disease. *J. Am. Coll. Cardiol.* 1994; 24: 546 – 54.

[5] Leone A. Cigarette smoking and health of the heart. *J. Roy. Soc. Health.* 1995; 115: 354 – 5.

[6] Glantz SA, Parmley WW. Passive smoking and heart disease. *JAMA.* 1995; 273: 1047 – 53.

[7] Kritz H, Schmid P, Sinzinger H. Passive smoking and cardiovascular risk. *Arch. Intern. Med.* 1995;155: 1942 – 8.

[8] Gray N. The social and economic implications of tobacco use. In: Proceedings of the Fifth World Conference on Smoking and Health, Forbes WF, Frecker RC, Nostbakken D eds., Canadian Council on Smoking and Health, Winnipeg, Canada, 1983; 77 – 92.

[9] Leone A. Cigarette smoking and cardiovascular damage: analytic review of the subject. *Singapore Med. J.* 1994; 35: 492 – 4.

[10] Asia and World Economy. The alternative engine. *The Economist,* Hong Kong, 18 October 2006.

[11] Hirayama T. Lung cancer in Japan: effects of nutrition and passive smoking. In: Mizell M, Correa P eds., *Lung cancer: Causes and Prevention. Verlag Chemie International, Deerfield Beach* (MA) 1984; 175 – 95.

[12] Garland C, Barret-Connor E, Suarez L, Criqui MH, Wingard DL. Effects of passive smoking on ischemic heart disease mortality of nonsmokers: a prospective study. *Am. J. Epidemiol.* 1985; 121: 645 – 50.

[13] Svendsen KH, Kuller LH, Martin MJ, Ockene JK. Effects of passive smoking in the Multiple Risk Factor Intervention Trial. *Am. J. Epidemiol.* 1987; 126: 783 – 95.

[14] Butler TL. The relationship of passive smoking to various health outcomes among Seventh-day Adventists in California (dissertation). Los Angeles, University of California, 1988.

[15] Helsing KJ, Sandler DP, Comstock GW, Chee E. Heart disease mortality in nonsmokers living with smokers. *Am. J. Epidemiol.* 1988; 127: 915 – 22.

[16] Hole DJ, Gillis CR, Chopra C, Hawthorne VM. Passive smoking and cardiorespiratory health in a general population in the west of Scotland. *BMJ.* 1989; 299: 423 – 7.

[17] Sandler DP, Comstock GW, Helsing KJ, Shore DL. Deaths from all causes in non-smokers who lived with smokers. *Am. J. Public Health.* 1989; 79: 163 – 7.

[18] Humble C, Croft J, Gerber A, Casper M, Hames CG, Tyroler HA. Passive smoking and 20-year cardiovascular disease mortality among nonsmoking wives, Evans County, Georgia. *Am. J. Public Health.* 1990; 80: 599 – 601.

[19] LeVois ME, Layard MW. Publication bias in the environmental tobacco smoke/coronary heart disease epidemiologic literature. *Regul. Toxicol. Pharmacol.* 1995; 21: 184 – 91.

[20] Stenland K, Thun M, Lally C, Heath C Jr. Environmental tobacco smoke and coronary heart disease in the American Cancer Society CPS-II cohort. *Circulation.* 1996; 94: 622 – 8.

[21] Kawachi I, Colditz GA, Speizer FE, Manson JE, Stampfer MJ, Willett WC, Hennekens CH. A prospective study of passive smoking and coronary heart disease. *Circulation.* 1997; 95: 2374 – 9.

[22] Steenland K. Passive smoking and the risk of the heart disease. *JAMA.* 1992; 267: 94 – 9.

[23] Dobson AJ, Alexander HM, Heller RF, Lloyd DM. Passive smoking and the risk of heart attack or coronary death. *Med. J. Aust.* 1991; 154: 793 – 7.

[24] Muscat JE, Wynder EL. Exposure to environmental tobacco smoke and the risk of heart attack. *Int. J. Epidemiol.* 1995; 24: 715 – 9.

[25] He Y, Lam TH, Li LS, Du RY, Jia GL, Huang JY, Zhang JS. Passive smoking at work as a risk factor for coronary heart disease in Chinese women who have never smoked. *BMJ.* 1994; 308: 380 – 4.

[26] Lee PN, Chamberlain J, Alderson MR. Relationship of passive smoking to risk of lung cancer and other smoking-associated diseases. *Br. J. Cancer.* 1986; 54: 97 – 105.

[27] He Y, Li LS, Wan ZH, Li LS, Zheng XL, Jia GL. Women's passive smoking and coronary heart disease. *Chinese J. Preventive Medicine.* 1989; 23: 19 – 22.

[28] Jackson R. The Auckland Heart Study: a case-control study of coronary heart disease (dissertation). Auckland University, New Zealand, 1989.

[29] La Vecchia C, D'Avanzo B, Franzosi MG, Tognoni G. Passive smoking and the risk of acute myocardial infarction. *Lancet.* 1993; 341:505 – 6.

[30] Layard MW. Ischemic heart disease and spousal smoking in the National Mortality Followback Survey. *Regulatory Toxicol and Pharmacol.* 1995; 21: 180 – 3.

[31] Tunstall-Pedoe H, Brown CA, Woodward M, Tavendale R. Passive smoking by self-report and serum cotinine and the prevalence of respiratory and coronary heart disease in the Scottish heart health study. *J. Epidemiol. Community Health.* 1995; 49: 139 – 43.

[32] Ciruzzi M, Pramparo P, Esteban O, Rozlosnik J, Tartaglione J, Abecasis B, César J, De Rosa J, Paterno C, Schargrodsky H. Case-control study of passive smoking at home and risk of acute myocardial infarction. *J. Am. Coll. Cardiol.* 1998;31: 797 – 803.

[33] McElduff P, Dobson AJ, Jackson R, Beaglehole R, Heller RF, Lay-Yee R. Coronary events and exposure to environmental tobacco smoke: a case-control study from Australia and New Zealand. *Tobacco Control.* 1998; 7: 41 – 6.

[34] Rosenlund M, Berglind N, Gustavsson A, Reuterwall C, Hallqvist J, Nyberg F, Pershangen G. Environmental tobacco smoke and myocardial infarction among never-smokers in the Stockholm Heart Epidemiolgy Program (SHEEP). *Epidemiology.* 2001; 12: 558 – 64.

[35] US Department of Health and Human Services . *The health consequences of smoking: A Report of the Surgeon General.* Atlanta: US Department of Health and Human Services, Centers for Disease Control and Prevention, National Center for Chronic Disease Prevention and Health Promotion, Office on Smoking and Health, 2004.

[36] Office of Environmental Health Hazard Assessment, California Environmental Protection Agency. Health effects of exposure to environmental tobacco smoke. *Final draft for scientific, public, and SRP review.* 1997; 8: 1 – 74.

[37] He Y, Lam TH, Li LS, Li LS, Du RY, Jia GL, Huang JY, Zhang JS. The number of coronary stenotic arteries and passive smoking exposure from husband in lifelong non-smoking women in Xi'an, China. *Atherosclerosis.* 1996; 127: 229 – 38.

[38] Sherman CB. Health effects of cigarette smoking. *Clin. Chest Med.* 1991; 12:643 – 58.

[39] Law MR, Morris JK, Wald NJ. Environmental tobacco smoke exposure and ischaemic heart disease: an evaluation of the evidence. *BMJ.* 1997; 315: 973 – 80.

[40] He J, Vupputuri S, Allen K, Prerost MR, Hughes J, Whelton PK. Passive smoking and the risk of coronary heart disease: a metanalysis of epidemiologic studies. *N. Engl. J. Med.* 1999; 340: 920 – 6.

[41] Thun M, Henley J, Apicella L. Epidemiologic studies on fatal and nonfatal cardiovascular disease and ETS exposure from spousal smoking. *EHP.* 1999, 107 (Suppl 6) : 841 – 6.

[42] Law MR, Hackshaw AK. Environmental tobacco smoke. *Br. Med. Bull.* 1996; 52: 22 – 34.

[43] Howard G, Burke GL, Szklo M, Tell GS, Eckfeldt J, Evans G, Heiss G. Active and passive smoking are associated with increased carotid wall thickness. *Arch. Intern. Med.* 1994; 154: 1277 – 82.

[44] Donnan GA, McNeil JJ, Adena MA, Doyle AE, O'Malley HM, Neill GC. Smoking as a risk factor for cerebral ischaemia. *Lancet.* 1989; 2: 643 – 7.

[45] Bonita R, Duncan J, Truelsen T, Jackson RT, Beaglehole R. Passive smoking as well as active smoking increases the risk of acute stroke. *Tobacco Control.* 1999; 8: 156 – 60.

[46] Howard G, Wagenknecht L, Cai J, CooperL, Kraut M, Toole JF. Cigarette smoking and other risk factors for silent cerebral infarction in the general population. *Stroke.* 1998b; 29: 913 – 7.

[47] You RX, Thrift AG, McNeil JJ, Davis SM, Donnan GA, and the Melbourne Stroke Risk Factor Study (MSRFS) Group. Ischemic stroke risk and passive exposure to spouses' cigarette smoking. *Am. J. Public Health.* 1999; 89: 572 – 5.

[48] Whincup PH, Gilg JA, Emberson JR, Jarvis MJ, Feyerabend C, Bryant A, Walker M, Cook DG. Passive smoking and risk of coronary heart disease and stroke: prospective study with cotinine measurement. *BMJ.* 2004; 329: 200 – 5.

[49] Howard J, Wagenknecht LE, Burke GL, Diez-Roux A, Evans GW, McGovern P, Nieto JF, Tell GS, for the ARIC Investigators. Cigarette smoking and progression of atherosclerosis; The atherosclerosis risk in communities (ARIC) study. *JAMA.* 1998; 279: 119 – 24.

[50] Werner RM, Pearson TA. What is so passive about passive smoking? Secondhand smoke as a cause of atherosclerotic disease. *JAMA.* 1998; 279: 157 – 8.

[51] Salonen JT, Salonen R. Ultrasonography assessed carotid morphology and risk of coronary heart disease. *Arterioscler. Thromb. Vasc. Biol.* 1991;11: 1245 – 9.

[52] Bots ML, Hoes AW, Koudstaal PJ, Hofman A, Grobbee DE. Common carotid intima-media thickness and risk of stroke and myocardial infarction: the Rotterdam Study. *Circulation.* 1997; 96: 1432 – 7.

Chapter 9

EXPERIMENTAL STUDIES

ABSTRACT

The analysis of different experimental studies conducted on both humans and animals undoubtedly show that exposure to passive smoking determines alterations for those structures like heart, arteries and cardiovascular metabolites that are usually negatively influenced by smoking compounds. Moreover, the lesions observed in animals are structural lesions that are always of the same type although of differing degrees. The latter is particularly related to the duration of the exposure rather than environmental concentration in toxics.

Endothelial cell permeability increase in size but not in number of atherosclerotic plaques. They also increase in arterial stiffness and perivascular infiltrates are the main artery changes described experimentally. The heart shows primarily changes which are related to coronary heart disease in both experimental human and animal studies. Lipid profile changes with reduced HDL-Cholesterol, platelet activation with increased adhesiveness and aggregation, increased fibrinogen levels are the other parameters which are shown to be altered in experimental findings on passive smoking.

Keywords: Experimental studies, human(s), animal(s), myocardium, coronary heart disease, endothelial dysfunction, exercise tolerance, arterial stiffness, lipid profile, platelet, fibrinogen.

In contrast with the observational studies on the epidemiology of cardiovascular damage from passive smoking exposure, which are usually large-scale studies with positive points of view, as well as with the limits already described, experimental studies often provide more reliable results since they primarily concern small samples of the studied population and set the goal to verify only those hypotheses of finding formulated by a single or a few group of researchers who personally follow the study. As a consequence of that, statistical estimates are conducted, in most cases, by greater care.

Some basic characteristics must be borne in mind to correctly assess an experimental finding particularly for those findings which are related to passive smoking exposure in an attempt to avoid misinterpretation of obtained results. That is even more necessary since opinions on the cardiovascular damage due to passive smoking exposure are, as often underlined, not yet unanimous. Therefore, it seems to be worthwhile to have a brief description of the requisite that supports the scientific significance of an experiment.

An experimental finding must follow (Figure 9.1) some essential rules: formulating an hypothesis of finding, complying with study design, identifying study material easily available since possible loss of information in the case of small samples can interfere with the reliability of the results, analyzing obtained results that enable one to accept totally or partially a formulated hypothesis or reject it completely.

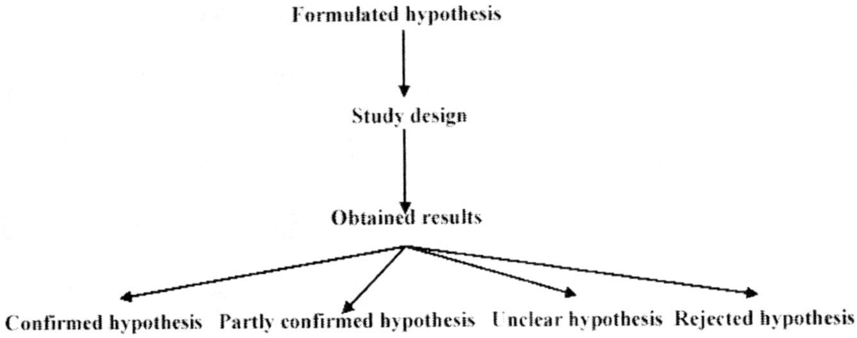

Figure 9.1. Characteristics of an experimental finding.

Firstly, formulated hypothesis must be relevant to the finding to be conducted, provide results that increase scientific knowledge, deal with outward opinions that are appropriate to the analyzing object, and particularly, always give reproducible data whenever experimental procedures act in the same way.

Study design must be addressed to verify formulated hypothesis in the best possible manner. It needs to be approved by both Ethic Committee and the enrolled population. Moreover, the enrolled population should be well prepared to reach the final steps of the study. If the study includes animals, obtained results require the capability to be translated to humans or living environments with a compatibility as great as it is possible.

Obtained results require to be easily interpreted, validated by a correct statistical estimate, be exactly reproducible by different researchers in different laboratories and particularly, verify formulated hypothesis. About that, results can fully confirm the hypothesis of the study, partly confirm it, give unclear conclusions which therefore would need further findings, and finally, reject the hypothesis. However the latter statement is not to be underestimated since it permits avoiding to formulate a new hypothesis by using those factors which can produce a type of result, the groundlessness of which has been well experimented.

Table 9.1 lists the main characteristics of an experimental finding as well as its addresses.

Table 9.1. Characteristics and addresses of an experimental study

Characteristic	Address
Formulated hypothesis	Relevant to finding, increasing scientific knowledge, giving reproducible results.
Study design	Verifying hypothesis, etic Committee and study population approval, animal result translation to humans.
Obtained results	Easy interpreting, statistically correct approach, reproducibility, confirm or rejection of the formulated hypothesis.

Experimental studies on the relationship between passive smoking exposure and cardiovascular damage which meet these characteristics can be considered as findings to be included among those which reach effective conclusions on the subject. It is therefore of basic importance that all the ways reached by carefully following the steps of Figure 9.1 are verified to warrant a scientific subject, as the damage from passive smoking exposure needs a strongly demonstrative support.

Findings may be conducted (Table 9.2.) through two ways with different characteristics: human findings following acute or chronic exposure, and animal findings with the same characteristics of exposure, although acute exposure is mainly used in experimental findings.

Table 9.2. Types of experimental studies on passive smoking exposure

Study material	Structure involved	Type of exposure
Experimental studies on humans	Heart	Acute
		Chronic
	Endothelium	Acute
		Chronic
Experimental animal studies	Myocardium	Acute
		Chronic
	Arteries	Acute
		Chronic

In the following sections, the main types of studies will be described with a particular attention to those which demonstrate, with no doubt, the harmful effects of exposure to passive smoking on both heart and blood vessels. Indeed, the studies which reach results experimentally showing relevant damage are significantly prevailing compared to those where the damage did not exist or, better yet, exist with scarce signs.

EXPERIMENTAL HUMAN STUDIES

Experimental human studies on the relationship between passive smoking exposure and cardiovascular system particularly point out functional disorders of the heart and blood vessels. These studies usually have been conducted after acute exposure to environmental tobacco smoke and such a condition well explains the type of alteration observed since, as it is already described, anatomical alterations in humans, which tend to appear a long time after the exposure.

Among functional parameters which have been tested in subjects acutely exposed to passive smoking, there are exercise tolerance and lipid profile either in healthy people or people with established ischemic heart disease. Functional disorders of the vessels have been mainly described for endothelial function associated with changes in platelet function and hemostatic metabolites (Table 9.3.).

Table 9.3. Main functional parameters tested experimentally in exposed subjects to passive smoking

Structure Involved	Tested Parameter
Heart	Exercise tolerance
Arteries	Endothelial function
Blood cells	Platelet function
Metabolites	Lipid profile
	Fibrinogen

Four studies analyzed exercise performance of healthy subjects and/or subjects with a previous heart disease [1–4], usually coronary heart disease. Exercise tolerance was investigated in the absence and in the presence of passive smoking exposure, with regard to carbon monoxide levels. Carbon monoxide is considered as the main toxic compound capable to negatively influence heart function. Its concentration during passive smoking exposure widely varied in the experimental findings, although it was maintained to a level of safety as well as to a concentration that may be easily met in public places.

In the study of Aronow [1], exercise performance of 10 men with stable exertional angina was evaluated. The men were exposed to environmental tobacco smoke twice: in a well-ventilated room, and in a room where ventilation was absent. Exposure to passive smoking induced heart rate, blood pressure and increase in carboxyhemoglobin concentration associated with a statistically significant decrease in angina threshold equal to 22% during exercise.

Pimm and coworkers [2] analyzed the response twice to exercise of 20 healthy young men and women: in an environment polluted by carbon monoxide to a concentration of 24 ppm and in an environment not polluted by carbon monoxide. Exercise on bicycle ergometer lasted 7 minutes. In a smoking environment study, people showed a significant increase in carboxyhemoglobin concentration which was not associated with any other disorder in functional cardiovascular parameters.

McMurray and coworkers [3] studied exercise performance of 8 young healthy men, who were 4 smokers and 4 nonsmokers, identifying a reduction in exercise duration in passive smoking environment as well as reduced maximal oxygen uptake. Increase in maximal respiratory exchange ratio, maximal blood lactate, ratings of perceived exertion, and ratio of ventilation to oxygen uptake was also observed, although with a statistical significance of p less than 0.05 and never more significant for each tested parameter.

Finally, Leone and coworkers [4] analyzed the effects of acute exposure to passive smoking of 9 healthy subjects and 10 subjects with a previous myocardial infarction who were tested and controlled since they performed the same bicycle ergometer exercise twice in a same environment: firstly, the environment was not polluted by carbon monoxide and then it was polluted by carbon monoxide at a concentration of 30 to 35 ppm. Analyzed parameters were: peak of exercise power, time to recovery of pre-exercise heart rate evaluated in minutes, levels of carboxyhemoglobin, and level of expired carbon monoxide. All studied subjects showed impaired exercise tolerance in a smoking environment, although with a different response. Healthy subjects only showed a statistically significant prolonged (p less tan 0.01) time to recovery of pre-exercise heart rate and increase in post-exercise carboxyhemoglobin concentrations. People suffering from a previous myocardial infarction had all the studied post-exercise parameters significantly impaired. Moreover, ischemic group showed a significantly higher incidence of ventricular arrhythmias during exercise in passive smoking environment [5] compared to that of the same subject performing the exercise in a smoke-free environment.

Table 9.4 summarizes the characteristics of a study population in the different findings as well as the response to exercise stress testing. Although differences in the types of populations and evaluated parameters existed, collected data concluded that a significant impairment in exercise performance was determined by exposure to carbon monoxide of passive smoking, especially for those people with established ischemic heart disease.

Table 9.4. Exercise tolerance in passive smoking and impaired parameters in passive smoking

Study	Population	Impaired Parameter
Aronow [1]	10 men with exertional angina	Increased heart rate
		Increased blood pressure
		Increased carboxyhemoglobin
		Reduced angina threshold
Pimm et al. [2]	20 healthy men and women	Increased carboxyhemoglobin
McMurray et al. [3]	8 healthy women	Reduced exercise duration
		Reduced maximal oxygen uptake
		Increased respiratory change ratio
		Increased blood lactate
		Increased perceived exertion rating
Leone et al. [4]	9 healthy people	Prolonged recovery pre-exercise heart rate
		Increased carboxyhemoglobin
	10 men with previous AMI	Prolonged recovery pre-exercise heart rate
		Reduction in peak of exercise power
		Increased carboxyhemoglobin
		Increased expired carbon monoxide
Leone et al. [5]	10 men with previous AMI	Ventricular arrhythmias

Abbreviations: AMI= acute myocardial infarction.

Finally, two further studies [6–7] on exercise tolerance of subjects with a history of coronary heart disease showed the appearance of signs of myocardial ischemia or ventricular arrhythmias when carbon monoxide existed in the environment where the exercise was performed.

Endothelial function is the vascular parameter particularly both clinically and experimentally investigated in nonsmokers exposed to passive smoking. As already described, endothelial dysfunction is considered to be an early event in the pathogenesis of the arterial plaque.

The response of the endothelium to environmental tobacco smoke exposure has been partly described in the Chapter 5 by the analysis of the paper of Celermajer and coworkers [8] published on "The New England Journal of Medicine" 1996. This finding demonstrated a significant impairment of the endothelial function following acute exposure to passive smoking with markedly altered flow-mediated brachial artery dilatation and no change in nitroglycerin dilatation response. Flow-mediated vasodilation is a parameter closely related to endothelial function. The impaired endothelium-dependent dilation was related to the dose of passive smoking. The authors suggested that environmental tobacco exposure, by affecting endothelial function, may damage the arterial intima even in young healthy adults.

Adverse vascular effects of environmental tobacco smoke may also be identified by experimentally studying aortic elasticity. Stefanidis and coworkers [9] investigated aortic elasticity in 48 male patients most of whom were suffering from coronary heart disease. By means of a sonometric catheter, the diameter of the aorta was measured, while simultaneously, arterial pressure at the same location was recorded. Passive smoking exposure reduced significantly aortic elasticity. Pathologically, stiffening of the aorta augments left ventricular afterload, thereby negatively affecting ventricular function. As tobacco causes coronary vasoconstrition [10–11], a stiffer aorta would worsen myocardial ischemia in those subjects suffering from coronary heart disease and among those with hypertension whose aortic distensibility is already compromised. Stefanidis and coworkers' finding tends to demonstrate that a double mechanism induces cardiovascular function impairment during passive smoking exposure: the one, a direct effect on the aortic elasticity, and another, an indirect effect involving coronary blood flow.

Changes in lipid profile and platelet function have been well identified experimentally after exposure to passive smoking. Highly significant in this context is the finding of Neufeld and coworkers [12]. Children of parents who smoked showed a mean lowering of HDL-Cholesterol equal to 11.2% when they were compared to children of nonsmoker relatives. This lowering in HDL-Cholesterol that was adjusted for potential confounders reduced its value to a significant 8.5% and is, by far, greater than that previously described in children. A prudential estimate of this data would be needed but there is clear evidence that exposed children may be affected negatively by passive smoking. Results of Neufeld and coworkers could feel the effects of high-risk lipid profiles of study population as well as other factors related to different lifestyles.

Lowering in HDL-Cholesterol might be due to the effect of nicotine on catecholamines levels [13].

Changes in lipid profile with a significant decrease in HDL-Cholesterol levels are reported by other studies [14–15] which also found high levels of cotinine and thiocyanate in children and pre-adolescents living together with smoking relatives.

The changes in lipid profile described in exposed children, compared to not exposed, are similar quantitatively to those observed between smoking children compared to nonsmoking children, although at a lower level. The reduction in HDL-Cholesterol in passive smokers may be mathematically estimated to be about two-thirds of that of active smokers. Mathematical procedures that permit to estimate the amount of decreased or increased parameter will be described in a new chapter of this book for what is concerning passive smoking exposure.

Among cell and metabolic parameters, platelet function and fibrinogen levels have been mainly analyzed under experimental conditions since they relate well to atherosclerotic plaque.

Experimental studies on platelets have been particularly conducted by a comparison of changes in platelet function between active smokers and nonsmokers. However, significant changes have been demonstrated in never smokers exposed to passive smoking. These changes have been evaluated by measuring platelet sensitivity to PGI2 [16–17]. Moreover, exposed smokers and nonsmokers to 20 minute passive smoking evidenced of interesting results. At baseline, and then before exposure, smokers showed a platelet activation greater than that of nonsmokers. After acute exposure, platelet activation in smokers was the same, while nonsmokers had a significant increase in platelet activation, that reached values almost similar to those of the platelets of smokers.

Studies on platelet activation after passive smoking exposure are mainly conducted by measurements of some chemicals that influence platelet function.

Nicotine would be the most important chemical in causing platelet adhesiveness and aggregation by both a direct role, and also inducing catecholamine release, although other smoking components may be involved in this mechanism.

Among coagulation metabolites, fibrinogen levels are strong predictors of risk for thrombosis [18–19]. Since fibrinogen levels increase in time, observational studies rather than experimental studies better show the negative effects of passive smoking on this parameter. Table 9.5 shows the main vascular, cell and metabolic parameters influenced negatively by passive smoking exposure under experimental conditions in humans.

Table 9.5. Vascular, cell, and metabolic parameters influenced experimentally by passive smoking in humans

Parameter	Response induced
Vascular endothelium	Impaired endothelial flow-mediated vasodilation
Aorta	Increase in stiffness
Lipid profile	Significant lowering in HDL-Cholesterol
Platelet function	Increased adhesiveness and aggregation
Fibrinogen	Increased thrombogenetic levels

From the analysis of experimental studies conducted in humans, there is clear evidence that exposure to passive smoking induces harmful effects on cardiovascular system which may be documented earlier and are also more aggressive than those of the observational studies. Such a fact is the consequence of the different study protocol between the two types of findings, which are expecting the occurrence of a negative event to be evaluated for observational studies, while experimental studies analyze the effects of damage from smoking at a scheduled time that is represented by the end of the experiment. Consequently, such a statement must be kept in mind when one gives an appraisal on the course of a phenomenon. However, experimental human studies on the negative effects of passive smoking exposure on cardiovascular system are complying with all the steps listed in Figure 9.1 and consequently, the conclusions reached provide reliable results about the certainty of the damage.

Experimental Animal Studies

An examination of the results obtained from experimental animal studies on the relationship between passive smoking exposure and cardiovascular system needs a preliminary statement. Alot of findings generically define exposure to cigarette smoking and what characterizes the type of exposure of the animal. There is often no clear explanation whether exposure to smoking is an active or passive exposure. Usually, experiments on animals are conducted in an environment polluted by cigarette smoke but not by the animal smoking a cigarette. Therefore, findings should be classified strictly as findings in passive smoking exposure, however, that does not always occur. By doing so, however, greater concentrations of smoking toxics could pollute the environment since studies on active smoking quantitatively require a major amount of chemicals. Moreover, chemicals may disperse into the environment and not be absorbed directly by exposed animals as active smoking would require. Even if we adjust the amount of pollutants to the body weight of the experimental animal, we find major concentrations of pollutants than those usually measured during passive smoking exposure, or lower concentrations, considering the type of exposure to active smoking. This type of experimental condition accelerates the progression of the lesions usually determined by passive smoking exposure, in the strict sense of the word, and aggravates their features. So, this is the main reason of the appearance of anatomical alterations which may be more rapidly documented in animal studies rather than in human studies, where functional disorders after acute exposure usually appear.

Exposure to passive smoking in experimental animal studies has demonstrated particularly alterations of great arteries and myocardium.

Among great arteries, lesions of the aorta and pulmonary artery have been described after acute, short-term exposure. In male New Zealand white rabbits maintained on a high cholesterol diet, accelerated atherosclerotic lesions of the aorta and pulmonary artery have been demonstrated [20]. Atherosclerosis progression would seem to be due to environmental tobacco smoke exposure but not to a major release of hormones by beta-adrenergic system since β-blocking drugs administered to animals did not protect against atherosclerosis progression from passive smoking, while the same drugs acted in decreasing the level of atherosclerosis not related to smoking exposure [21].

In another study [22], growing of pre-existing atherosclerotic plaques was induced in cockerels exposed to environmental tobacco smoke when exposed animals were compared to those not exposed. Moreover, the total number of atherosclerotic plaques did not change after passive smoking inhalation but a significant increase in plaque size was observed. Growing did not seem to depend on the level of passive smoking chemicals since it was seen also with lower chemical concentration in the environment [23].

Carbon monoxide is the main component of passive smoking, capable to induce experimental changes in animals. Astrup [24] found that carbon monoxide increased endothelial membrane permeability. Electron microscopic investigations confirmed this observation. Rabbits exposed to a mixture of carbon monoxide developed arterial lesions resulting in a considerable accumulation of lipids similarly to what was documented by Sarma and coworkers [25] in human coronary artery exposed to carbon monoxide " in vitro". Increased coronary blood flow [26–28] is the response of the heart to mild carbon monoxide exposure although, in these circumstances, there is an increase of carboxyhemoglobin. Such a behavior has been documented experimentally in both humans and dogs. Moreover, dogs should show pathological changes in the heart after long-term exposure to high carbon monoxide concentrations [29–32]. In a large majority of observations, electrocardiographic, but not gross changes were seen. Also myocardial microscopic changes were found [29].

Similarly, findings on different animals showed electrocardiographic changes after carbon monoxide exposure [33].

Notwithstanding the structural alterations what have been described, it is very hard to identify the cardiotoxic levels of tobacco exposure at which animals must be maintained to show repeatable lesions. It is no doubt that these levels are determined experimentally, but since a lot of chemical compounds are present in environmental tobacco smoke with often different concentrations, it could be that when a stably dosed concentration of a metabolite is reached, the other toxic compounds could measure concentrations already harmful for the experiment or otherwise be underdosed with no possibility to potentiate the degree of damage of the exposed animal. Therefore, experiments conducted simply measure the concentrations of those metabolites like nicotine and carbon monoxide that are recognized to be more toxic for cardiovascular system with no interest in assessing the exact levels necessary to induce repeatable lesions.

Three types of lesions may have been documented in experimental animal studies after exposure to passive smoking: gross changes, which are hard to identify after single acute exposure, evident histologic changes, and ultrastructural changes. These last two may have been observed earlier.

Main changes described in experimental animal studies as well as the type of alterations observed are summarized in Table 9.6.

Table 9.6. Cardiovascular changes described in experimental animal studies after exposure to passive smoking

Structure Involved	Type of alterations
Arteries	Endothelial cell permeability increase
	Increase in size but not in number of atherosclerotic plaque
	Increased arterial stiffness
	Perivascular infiltrates
Heart	Myocardial necrosis
	Increased infarct size
	Focal myocardial hemorrhage
	Fibrosis
	Electrocardiographic changes
	Myocardial fiber swelling
	Mitochondrial changes
	Ribosome changes
Lipid profile	LDL accumulation in perfused carotid arteries

Among ultrastructural changes, degenerative changes of mitochondria with edema, external membrane lesion and swelling have been described by Thomsen and Kjeldsen [34] to the myocardium of guinea pigs after prolonged inhalation of cigarette smoking, lasting at least 12 weeks. These alterations were similar to those described by Cantin and Leone [35] in myocardial cells of animals with experimental myocardial infarction induced by different techniques but not smoking. Such an evidence would focus the severity of the alterations determined by passive smoking exposure. Lough also [36] described similar alterations to myocardial mitochondria of guinea pigs exposed to the smoke of 8 cigarettes a day for 15 weeks. Author also found increased lipid content in mitochondria as well as enhanced autophagolysosomal activity due to carbon monoxide. Kjeldsen and coworkers [37] concluded that in experimental animal studies, ultrastructural alterations to myocardium that were seen after prolonged smoking exposure were similar to those showed in myocardial damage of rabbits exposed to carbon monoxide that are usually characterized by more evident myocardial fibrosis. Fibrosis could be, pathogenetically, the result of a chronic and repeated cardiac harm for prolonged exposure that would cause lesions progressively and in different stages.

Exposure to environmental tobacco smoke has been demonstrated to be capable of increasing myocardial infarct size in a Sprague-Dawley rat model of ischemia and reperfusion [38].

Finally, in Sprague-Dawley rats, acute exposure to passive smoking increased LDL accumulation in perfused carotid arteries, also after only a single exposure [39].

Experimental animal studies are, without a doubt, the clearest evidence of the harmful effect on cardiovascular system as a consequence of passive smoking exposure. Athough exposed animals do not always reach the same number or level of lesions after exposure, there is constant evidence that structural damage exists and always with the same characteristics. Moreover, also experimentally involved structures are those usually affected by the harmful effects that exposure to passive smoking may determine on humans.

References

[1] Aronow WS. Effect of passive smoking on angina pectoris. *N. Engl. J. Med.* 1978; 299: 21 – 4.

[2] Pimm PE, Silverman F, Shepard RJ. Physiological effects of acute passive exposure to cigarette smoke. *Arch. Environ. Health.* 1978; 33: 201 – 13.

[3] McMurray RG, Hicks LL, Thompson DL. The effects of passive inhalation of cigarette smoke on exercise performance. *Eur. J. Appl. Physiol.* 1985; 54: 196 – 200.

[4] Leone A, Mori L, Bertanelli F, Fabiano P, Filippelli M. Indoor passive smoking: Its effect on cardiac performance. *Int. J. Cardiol.* 1991; 33: 247 – 52.

[5] Leone A, Bertanelli F, Mori L, Fabiano P, Bertoncini G. Ventricular arrhythmias by passive smoke in patients with pre-existing myocardial infarction. *J. Am. Coll. Cardiol.* 1992; 3: 256 A.

[6] Allred EN, Blecker ER, Chaitman BR, Dahms TE, Gottlieb SO, Hackney JD, Pagano M, Selvester RH, Walden SM, Warren J. Short-term effects of carbon monoxide exposure on the exercise performance of subjects with coronary artery disease. *N. Engl. J. Med.* 1989; 321: 1426 – 32.

[7] Sheps DS, Herbst MC, Hinderliter AL, Adams KF, Ekeland LG, O'Neil JJ, Goldstein GM, Brombey PA, Dalton JL, Ballenger MN, Davis SM, Kooch GG. Production of arrhythmias by elevated carboxyhemoglobin in patients with coronary artery disease. *Ann. Intern. Med.* 1990; 113: 343 – 51.

[8] Celermajer DS, Adams MR, Clarkson P, Robinson J, McCredie R, Donald A, Deanfield JE. Passive smoking and impaired endothelium-dependent arterial dilatation in healthy young adults. *N. Engl. J. Med.* 1996; 334: 150 – 4.

[9] Stefanidis C, Vlachopoulos C, Tsiamis E. Unfavorable effects of passive smoking in aortic function in men. *Ann. Intern. Med.* 1998; 128: 426 – 34.

[10] Moreyra AE, Lacy CR, Wilson AC, Kumar A, Kostis JB. Arterial blood nicotine concentration and coronary vasoconstrictive effect of low-nicotine cigarette smoking. *Am. Heart J.* 1992; 124: 392 – 7.

[11] Quillen JE, Rossen JD, Oskarsson HJ, Minor RL Jr, Lopez AG, Winniford MD. Acute effect of cigarette smoking on the coronary circulation constriction of epicardial and resistance vessels. *J. Am. Coll. Cardiol.* 1993; 22: 642 – 7.

[12] Neufeld EJ, Mietus-Snyder M, Beiser AS, Baker AL, Newburger JW. Passive cigarette smoking and reduced HDL cholesterol levels in children with high-risk lipid profiles. *Circulation.* 1997; 96: 1403 – 7.

[13] Anthony HM. Reactive changes in the blood of smokers and the development of arterial diseases and COPD, A review: Evidence of associations between changes and subsequent disease with implications for the evaluation of harmful effects of cigarettes and for susceptibility to the chronic effects of inhaled pollutants. *Rev. Environ. Health.* 1989; 8: 25 – 86.

[14] Moskowitz WB, Mosteller M, Schieken RM, Bossano R, Hewitt JK, Bodurtha JN, Segrest JP. Lipoprotein and oxygen transport alterations in passive smoking preadolescent children. *Circulation.* 1990; 81: 586 – 92.

[15] Feldman J, Shenker IR, Etzel RA, Spierto FW, Liliefield DE, Nussbaum M, Jacobson MS. Passive smoking alters lipid profiles in adolescents. *Pediatrics.* 1991; 88: 259 – 64.

[16] Sinzinger H, Kefalides A. Passive smoking severely decreases platelet sensitivity to antiaggregatory prostaglandins. *Lancet.* 1982; 2: 392 – 3.

[17] Burghuber OC, Punzengruber C, Sinzinger H, Haber P, Silberbauer K. Platelet sensitivity to prostacyclin in smokers and nonsmokers. *Chest.* 1986; 90: 34 –38.

[18] Kannel WB, D'Agostino RB, Belanger AJ. Fibrinogen, cigarette smoking, and risk of cardiovascular disease: insights from the Framingham Study. *Am. Heart J.* 1987; 113: 1006 – 10.

[19] Meade TW, Imeson JD, Stirling Y. Effects of changes in smoking and other characteristics on clotting factors and the risk of ischaemic heart disease. *Lancet.* 1987; 2: 986 – 8.

[20] Zhu B-Q, Sun Y-P, Sievers RE, Isenberg WM, Glantz SA, Parmley WW. Passive smoking increases experimental atherosclerosis in cholesterol-fed rabbits. *J. Am. Coll. Cardiol.* 1993; 21: 225 – 32.

[21] Sun Y-P, Zhu B-Q, Sievers RE, Glantz SA, Parmley WW. Metoprolol does not attenuate atherosclerosis in lipid-fed rabbits exposed to environmental tobacco smoke. *Circulation* 1994; 89: 2260 – 5.

[22] Penn A, Snyder CA. Inhalation of sidestream cigarette smoke accelerates development of arteriosclerotic plaques. *Circulation.* 1993; 88: 1820 – 5.

[23] Penn A, Chen L-C, Snyder CA. Inhalation of steady-state sidestream smoke from one cigarette promotes arteriosclerotic plaque development. *Circulation.* 1994; 90: 1363 – 7.

[24] Astrup P. Some physiological and pathological effects of moderate carbon monoxide exposure. *BMJ.* 1972; 4: 447 – 52.

[25] Sarma JSM, Tillmans H, Ikeda S, Bins RJ. The effect of carbon monoxide on lipid metabolism of human coronary arteries. *Atherosclerosis.* 1975; 22: 193 – 8.

[26] Permutt S, Fahri L. Tissue hypoxia and carbon monoxide. In: *Effects of chronic exposure to low levels of carbon monoxide on human health, behaviour, and performance*. National Academy of Sciences, National Academy of Engineering, Washington, DC, 1969; 18 – 24.

[27] Adams JD, Erickson HH, Stone HL. Myocardial metabolism during exposure carbon monoxide in the conscious dog. *J. appl. Physiol.* 1973; 34: 238 – 42.

[28] Horwath SM, Raven PB, Dahms TE, Gray DJ. Maximal aerobic capacity at different levels of carboxyhemoglobin. *J. appl. Physiol.* 1975; 38: 300 – 3.

[29] Lindenberg R, Preziosi T, Levy D, Christensen MH. Experimental investigation of carbon monoxide toxicity. Air Pollution Medical Research Conference, Los Angeles, CA, 1961.

[30] Preziosi T, Lindenberg R, Levy D, Christenson M. An experimental investigation in animals of the functional and morphological effects of single and repeated exposures to high and low concentrations of carbon monoxide. *Ann. NY Acad. Sci.* 1970; 174: 369 – 84.

[31] Lewey FH, Drabkin DD. Experimental chronic carbon monoxide poisoning of dogs. *Am. J. Med. Sci.* 1944; 208: 502 – 11.

[32] Ehrich WE, Bellet S, Lewey FH. Cardiac changes from CO poisoning. *Am. J. Med. Sci.* 1944; 208: 512 – 23.

[33] DeBias DA, Banerjee CM, Birkhead NC, Harrer WV, Kazal LA. Carbon monoxide inhalation effects following myocardial infarction in monkeys. *Arch. Environ. Health.* 1973; 27: 161 – 7.

[34] Thomsen HK, Kjeldsen K. Threshold limit for carbon monoxide-induced myocardial damage. *Arch. Environ. Health.* 1974; 29: 73 – 8.

[35] Cantin M, Leone A. Morphology of myocardial infarction. *Meth. Achiev. Exp. Pathol.* 1981; 10: 244 – 84.

[36] Lough J. Cardiomyopathy produced by cigarette smoke. Ultrastructural observations in guinea pigs. *Arch. Pathol. Lab. Med.* 1978; 102: 377 – 80.

[37] Kjeldsen K, Thomsen HK, Astrup P. Effects of carbon monoxide on myocardium. Ultrastructural changes in rabbits after moderate, chronic exposure. *Circ. Res.* 1974;34: 339 – 48.

[38] Zhu BQ, Sun JP, Sievers R, Glantz SA, Parmley WW, Wolfe CL. Exposure to environmental tobacco smoke increases myocardial infarct size in rats. *Circulation.* 1994; 89: 1282 – 90.

[39] Roberts KA, Rezai AA, Pinkerton KE, Rutledge JC. Effect of environmental tobacco smoke on LDL accumulation in the artery wall. *Circulation.* 1996; 94: 2248 – 53.

Chapter 10

DAMAGE FOR SPECIAL CATEGORIES

ABSTRACT

Special categories of subjects like women, children and adolescents, and old subjects can respond to passive smoking exposure for what is concerning the cardiovascular system in a different way with regard to the type of exposed men's response.

Such a fact seems to be related particularly to the physiological status that accompanies the gender and different phases of age. Moreover, since similar lesions are sometimes the consequence of either passive smoking exposure or individual "constellation", it is hard to establish exactly what belongs to one condition rather than the other.

Pre-menopausal women may usually be protected by the harmful effects of passive smoking by their endocrine constellation, unless, at the same time, they assume oral contraceptive drugs. The latter condition makes woman susceptible to be affected by thrombogenic events since the association between smoking and contraception induces a phenomena of hypercoagulability. On the contrary, post-menopausal woman loses the estrogen protection and therefore may be affected negatively by passive smoking exposure in a way similar to that observed in men. In post-menopause, therefore, possible thrombotic events in women are due to a type of atherogenetic but not thrombogenic response. Pregnant woman, according to a very recent report, would have an increased incidence up to 30% to bear children affected by congenital heart disease.

Child cardiovascular system is at birth regulated on a sympathetic attitude with elevated heart rate and often intolerance to the exercise. Therefore, exposure of cardiovascular system to passive smoking is particularly harmful in children and infants.

Finally, elderly makes difficult to recognize those cardiovascular alterations caused by passive smoking exposure rather than those caused by other major risk factors, being the alterations induced by both almost similar, factors and characterized by increased arterial stiffness and presence of atherosclerotic plaques. Moreover, changes determined by other major coronary risk factors like combined systolic and diastolic hypertension and diabetes mellitus are usually more harmful than those caused by passive smoking exposure or high cholesterol levels in aged individuals. However, reports underline a significantly major incidence of coronary heart disease and stroke in old subjects exposed chronically to passive smoking.

Keywords: Passive smoking , pre-menopausal woman, post-menopausal woman, pregnancy, children, sympathetic attitude, elderly, arterial stiffness, vagal tone.

As one can deduce from reading the previous chapters, the type of cardiovascular damage caused by exposure to passive smoking usually follows some characteristics which permit to identify either the mechanism by which it occurs or the body structures particularly involved. Notwithstanding that, assessing the type of cardiovascular damage from passive smoking has been wrongly overlooked in many findings. On the contrary, my opinion is that its recording and understanding allows us to interpret all those pathologic data associated with smoking exposure as well as the different characteristics which may be related to special categories of exposed individuals. It is well known that children, adolescents, aged subjects and, in some cases, premenopausal or postmenopausal women, may respond differently to smoking exposure according to the functional characteristics of cardiovascular system due to intrinsic constitutional properties.

TYPE OF CARDIOVASCULAR DAMAGE

Four types of cardiovascular damage (Table 10.1.) are a consequence of acute or chronic exposure to passive smoking: a functional damage, that usually involves acute exposure; a clinical damage that is often observed to follow chronic exposure or acute exposure of subjects chronically exposed; an anatomical damage that is typical of the chronic exposure or acute exposure, within certain limits, of animals studied experimentally; and a different combination of the above damages.

Table 10.1. Type of cardiovascular damage and its characteristic

Type of damage	Exposure	Characteristic
Functional damage	Acute exposure	Functional disorders; no anatomical alteration.
Clinical damage	Chronic exposure or acute exposure of chronically exposed	Functional disorders and symptoms of heart disease.
Anatomical damage	Chronic exposure or acute exposure in animal experiment	Structural alterations of different degree.
Combined damage	Both acute and chronic exposure	All types of alterations differently combined.

Functional damage, usually following an acute exposure to passive smoking, is in the first phases of exposure, transient and recognizes autonomic system involvement as a main pathogenetic factor [1 – 4]. Some parameters rather than others are negatively influenced by functional damage. This is what it is about altered responses: heart rate and systolic blood pressure usually increased, exercise tolerance usually impaired, and cardiac rhythm disorders. All these disorders are functional changes which are also maintained by the increased catecholamine levels usually associated with acute passive smoking exposure. Functional damage is specifically harmful for those subjects who suffer from ischemic heart disease as well as for those who are chronically exposed to passive smoking, being autonomic system and catecholamine release factors, in themselves, capable to cause spontaneously detrimental effects on both heart and blood vessels.

Clinical damage affects primarily those individuals who are customary exposed to passive smoking everywhere, but particularly in homes and workplaces. Symptoms referable to angina pectoris, myocardial infarction, arrhythmias and respiratory disease [5-6] may be worsened when this type of damage exists. A concomitant established anatomical damage, that acts as an underlying disease, is often associated with clinical damage. Also the association with a transiently functional damage, that may appear after acute environmental tobacco smoke exposure of subjects chronically exposed, worsens clinical damage of those individuals with symptoms related to coronary and cerebrovascular disease.

Anatomical damage is the final and unavoidable result of chronic and prolonged exposure to passive smoking. Its development is usually late but progressive until it reaches the characteristics of irreversibility. Stable alterations that are associated with an anatomical damage more often involve coronary arteries, systemic arteries causing hypertension and cerebrovascular disease, and myocardium [7 – 9]. In several cases, anatomical alterations support or aggravate pre-existing clinical symptoms. Impairment of clinical symptoms in individuals chronically exposed to passive smoking could be a useful, even if indirect, sign to follow-up furtherly worsening and progression of underlying anatomical damage.

Different experimental studies examined in the previous chapters would demonstrate undoubtedly that carbon monoxide plays a pivotal role in causing, maintaining and worsening anatomical damage. Levels of carboxyhemoglobin over 1.41% seem to be the concentrations of the metabolite that could chronically activate the impairment of cardiovascular system.

The main factor to support anatomical damage is the progression of an atherosclerosis lesion that can be triggered by a functional damage causing endothelial dysfunction, platelet function changes and altered fibrinogen levels. As one can see, all those factors capable of determining cardiovascular alterations from passive smoking are involved in the causative mechanism of the anatomical damage, which is the absolute final and heaviest result of passive smoking exposure. Anatomical damage may then be followed by those complications that induce severe and, sometimes fatal, cardiovascular events.

A cause-effect link would regulate, therefore, anatomical damage and passive smoking exposure, leading to consider environmental tobacco smoke as more than a simple cardiovascular risk factor but an etiologic factor of disease. However, this pattern will be better discussed in the next chapter.

Once the type of damage has been identified, there is need to assess how it can damage cardiovascular system of subjects different for gender and age who may respond differently to smoking exposure.

Women and Passive Smoking

In my opinion, some interesting considerations should be carried out to establish the exact relationship between environmental tobacco smoke and female gender.

Some types of responses of woman to passive smoking exposure have been analyzed in Chapter 6. Here, we believe it to be useful to underline the characteristics of heart and blood vessel damage that can be deduced by the different reports of epidemiological studies of women exposed to passive smoking, not only at home but also in workplaces. The risk for cardiovascular events in women differs from that in men because of, as already reported, sexual hormone constellation that seems to protect pre-menopausal woman from heart attacks, whereas that does not occur for post-menopausal woman. So, cardiovascular risk of woman of some age is lower than that of man, whereas in some age it appears to be equal or, even greater, than that in man.

A critical question, yet with no clear answer, is: why and how does a woman's endocrine constellation protect from the major nonfatal and fatal coronary events whereas this protection falls in presence of contraceptive use or post-menopause? Indeed, contraceptive drugs tend to maintain women in a premenopausal status but they do not protect woman.

An indirect answer to the above question that could also explain the difference in response with men at different ages is due to the type of changes of woman who use oral contraceptions and simultaneously smoke [10]. Oral contraceptives, particularly combined with smoke, can cause a state of increased coagulability usually potentiated by cigarette smoke, and that induces more easily thrombi formation. That does not occur if the two factors, smoking and oral contraceptive drugs, are not associated. Then, the response in pre-menopausal woman is not of a atherosclerotic type but of a thrombogenic type. On the contrary, since hormone constellation lowers in post-menopausal woman, she has a response of atherogenic type, similar to that in men, to smoking exposure instead of a thrombogenic type. The difference in the two types of responses are of basic importance, because the atherogenic response to smoking is due only to exposure of the woman, whereas the thrombogenic response usually needs woman exposure added to another factor, specifically oral contraceptive use. That leads to an increase in cardiovascular risk as well as to a type of response different than that observed in men.

There is evidence that both functional and structural disorders observed in the type of cardiovascular damage in never smoker women exposed to passive smoking, lead in a large majority to symptoms related to ischemic heart disease or cerebrovascular disease [11 – 20]. Such a fact would be furtherly indirect but a significant confirmation that women exposed to passive smoking could have a progression of atherosclerotic lesions, the increase of which is potentiated also by the higher systolic and diastolic blood pressure observed when women lived in a home polluted by environmental tobacco smoke. Therefore, exposure of nonsmoker women to passive smoking cannot be regarded as a safe involuntary habit.

Pregnant woman exposed to passive smoking seems to be at risk to bear children with a higher incidence of congenital cardiopathies present at birth. Exposure to two or more current household smokers [21] was associated with reduced mean mid expiratory flow and forced expiratory flow, which are parameters investigating mainly lung function, but also indirectly, cardiopulmonary function. However, after adjustment for in utero exposure, deficit in above parameters, although present, was not statistically significant. Other findings [22] could establish that exposure to passive smoking during pregnancy is an independent risk factor for low birth weight, sudden infant death syndrome [23], and congenital heart defects [24]. The latter report experienced that maternal smoking and tobacco exposure during pregnancy were associated with a significantly increased risk of congenital heart disease, especially septal and right-sided obstructive defects. In an interview of the main author of the paper reported by the "Chicago Tribune" [25], he affirmed that smoking cigarette just before becoming pregnant and shortly thereafter could increase woman's risk of having a baby with a congenital heart defect by 60% to 80%. And women who are exposed to environmental tobacco smoke at home or workplaces increased their risk by 30% of bearing infants with congenital heart disease.

Therefore, a pregnant woman's exposure to passive smoking can harm her fetus and the effects of damage are compounded when the child is exposed to passive smoking after birth.

Table 10.2. summarizes the different responses of woman to passive smoking exposure with regard to her physiologic status.

Table 10.2. Responses of a woman to passive smoking with regard to her physiological status

Physiological status	Main responses
Pre-menopause	Protection against passive smoking
Pre-menopause+ oral contraceptive	Thrombogenic response (hypercoagulability)
Post-menopause	Atherogenic response (lipid accumulation)
Pregnancy	Congenital heart defect increase Cardiopulmonary function impairment Sudden infant death syndrome

As one can see, female gender meets different phases during her life and these occurences are associated with possibly different physiological patterns of response to environmental tobacco smoke exposure. Moreover, it should be kept in mind that the different phases which characterize a woman's life are not strictly schematic existing transition periods which may determine a mosaic of intermediate responses, which are hard to interpret when we analyze the exposure to passive smoking.

Children and Passive Smoking

Also children exposure to passive smoking is worthwhile to be analyzed separately since the characteristics of the exposure and type of response evoked may be different from those observed in men and follow a way related to the functional characteristic of cardiovascular system in infancy. Moreover, observed results could be susceptible of inaccuracies because they derive in a large majority from parental interviews, which may give information bias [26–27].

It is useful, therefore, to describe the main differences in responses, observed physiologically from the of cardiovascular system of children compared to those of adults, to better interpret those alterations which may be related to passive smoking exposure.

At birth, cardiovascular system undergoes those progressive changes that will be for an adult heart. Therefore, in children there are some characteristics that may be considered as an advantage with regard to the adult heart and, on the contrary, others that predispose child cardiovascular system more heavily to harmful effects of passive smoking exposure.

Initially child heart rate is considerably more elevated than that of adults. Such a factor is accompanied by an autonomic system response that differs from that of the adults since adults usually have a balanced autonomic system function. On the contrary, a sympathetic attitude of cardiovascular system is prevailing in children and pre-adolescent. This type of physiological status makes cardiovascular system susceptible of a major degree of damage from passive smoking exposure since, as just described, all those conditions that determine an hyperfunction of autonomic system. In some cases, increased catecholamine release potentiate the harmful effects of exposure to smoking. Moreover, an increased condition of emotional stress, peculiar of infancy, may sometimes induce exercise intolerance in children. By these factors, which negatively influence the response of cardiovascular system to passive smoking exposure, there are others with effects that may reduce the harm from exposure to smoking: a usual absence of other major cardiovascular risk factors, unless a familial history of ischemic heart disease, is the absence of atherosclerotic lesions, even if fatty streaks may be seen early in artery vessels of children and adolescents, and a diet with a prevalence of proteins and vitamins necessary for an optimal growing of young children. It is known that particularly some vitamins can hinder the negative effects of smoking. Table 10.3. lists positive and negative factors that may be observed in children exposed to passive smoking.

Table 10.3. Positive and negative factors that influence passive smoking exposure in children

Positive factors	Negative factors
Absence of major cardiovascular risk factors	Sympathetic tone and catecholamine increase
Absence of atherosclerotic plaques	Possible exercise intolerance
Diet rich in proteins and vitamins	Emotional stress state

For the aforesaid reasons, children who are exposed to passive smoking are suffering particularly from respiratory simptoms [28] more than cardiovascular symptoms. Among respiratory symptoms, asthma and respiratory infections [29] are prevailing in children of parents who smoke compared to those living with nonsmoker parents. Moreover, there is a significant relationship between the incidence of respiratory diseases and the number of cigarettes smoked indoors. However, such an occurence also characterizes cardiovascular alterations due to indoor passive smoking exposure of children.

Since environmental tobacco smoke primarily causes those alterations of the heart and blood vessels which are closely related to a progression of the atherosclerosis, the main pathological characteristic of which is plaque formation, it is easy to recognize the reasons of the reduced impairment of cardiovascular system in children where atherosclerosis is usually far from developing due to the fact of the youngest age of this category of subjects. From examining Table 10.3, one can see that a reduced power of both those factors having a protective effect on the damage induced by passive smoking exposure, namely absence of atherosclerotic plaque and the major cardiovascular risk factors, similarly to what occurs especially in adults, negative exposure to passive smoking. Moreover, doubts exist about the scientific reliability of those data that have been collected via parents' questionnaire using merely general questions such as the presence or absence of smokers in the household, the exact number of cigarettes smoked, socio-economic condition and education, and characteristics of indoor spaces where children live. However, children exposed to tobacco smoke [27] have been distinguished, and could be distinguished, from non-exposed people by the measurements of urinary cotinine concentrations. As described in a previous chapter (see chapter 2), measuring urinary concentrations of cotinine should be an effective method to assess involuntary smoking exposure, but it may be used in a limited number of subjects, since there are heavy difficulties to dose the bio-metabolite on a large-scale. However, exposure of children to environmental tobacco smoke must be avoided due to the consistent increase in cardiovascular risk identified in adults.

ELDERLY AND PASSIVE SMOKING

Aged subjects need some considerations to be done for assessing the real result of their exposure to passive smoking as well as the type of cardiovascular damage which may be caused by the exposure.

It is necessary to premise that heart disease is a common occurence of the elderly and some anatomo-functional characteristics related to elderly may produce confusion in interpreting which alterations are due to passive smoking exposure or to advanced age, being the type of alterations similar in a large number of cases. Moreover, heart and cerebrovascular disease is the major cause of mortality and morbidity in 65 and older age people [30].

Besides, assessment of cardiovascular risk factors is pertinent even in elderly subjects, being a history of hypertension or diabetes mellitus usually associated with increased risk of atherosclerosis, which characterizes the older age with a different degree of alterations, whereas smoking, elevated cholesterol concentrations, factors that together can induce heavily atherosclerotic plaque formation, and family history of cardiovascular disease appear to have much less significance [31]. Moreover, a previous study [32] demonstrated that poor prognosis of elderly patients with a previous myocardial infarction was not related to age but to gender and the type of coronary risk factors. Among these factors, systolic hypertension was the most frequent factor to appear with no negative prognostic significance, unless it was associated with diabetes mellitus or concomitant diastolic hypertension.

Under statistical pattern, when one analyzes the different cardiovascular risks, including, among these factors, the age of the subjects by using Student's test (see also chapter 7), there will be the possibility that each factor separately could reveal a statistical significance. Instead, by using those statistical methods, which compare the statistical significance of different risk factors – and correctly use the latter tests, a very interesting observation arises: in elderly patients, each factor could induce changes in the functions of the cardiovascular system, but in any case, there will be a clear prevailing effect of some of them rather than others and therefore, it is very difficult to establish what alterations belong to what factor. Moreover, all the alterations that one can observe as an effect of a single risk factor relate well to the characteristics of the damage caused by other factors. Moreover, exposure duration becomes more and more complicated damage interpretation, since even if exposure to passive smoking last for a long time, there is no evidence of what has produced the alterations, being themselves the final way, as aforesaid, of several factor effects.

Another more important problem is to define the age to which an individual should be considered as an elderly subject. Unfortunately, there is no specific biological determinant of a physiological age that can be applied appropriately to different individuals and therefore, this parameter is often based on physical appearance. However, the old people are, conventionally, those subjects over 65 years old.

Cardiovascular system in elderly usually responds to passive smoking exposure in a manner that may be different from that of men without advanced age.

Autonomic nervous system, a structure influenced negatively by the exposure to passive smoking, feels the effects of aging. Primarily, phasic variation in heart rate accompanying respiration is attenuate with increasing age as a consequence of diminished vagal activity [33]. Also the sensitivity of baroreceptor reflex in elderly is impaired with an evident decrease in its function [34–35]. The baroreceptors are located in the wall of the aorta and respond to deformation of the wall. The decrease in sensitivity of baroceptors would be mainly due to an increased aortic stiffness. On the contrary, carotid sinus hypersensitivity may be increased [36–37]. Such a response is unclear and therefore, it needs further investigations.

The effects of aging on β-adrenergic system have also been examined by an experimental study [38]. It has been demonstrated that the amount of isoproterenol, a chemical compound capable to increase heart rate significantly, which needed to increase heart rate of 25 beats per minute increased with increasing age and concomitantly, the amount of propranolol necessary to block the heart rate response decreased with increasing age. Thus, β-adrenergic system appeared to be less sensitive to both agonist and antagonist drugs with a sensible imbalance in observed responses. A similar decreased sensitivity has been noted for the inotropic response to catecholamines [30]. This reduced sensitivity seemed to be related to catecholamine receptors that were unable to respond physiologically to the binding of a chemical substance with the receptor.

As one can deduce, the different autonomic response in elderly compared to that of younger individuals may determine a misinterpretation of the alterations observed in old individuals who had been exposed to passive smoking. Table 10.4 compares the responses of some parameters to passive smoking exposure and the responses of the same parameters observed in the elderly.

Table 10.4. Comparison of the responses of autonomic and adrenergic system to passive smoke exposure in adults and in the elderly

Passive smoking	Elderly
Increased heart rate (increased sympathetic tone)	Increased heart rate (reduced vagal tone)
Arterial stiffness increase	Arterial stiffness increase
Increased response to catecholamines	Altered response to catecholamines
Increased inotropic response	Altered inotropic response
Atherosclerotic plaque formation	Presence of atherosclerotic plaques
Endothelial dysfunction	Impaired endothelium response

As Table 10.4. clearly shows, some changes in the elderly are almost similar to that caused by passive smoking exposure in adults. Moreover, some other responses well defined after passive smoking exposure, particularly increase in inotropic response and endothelial dysfunction are not easily interpretable in the elderly, and that does not clarify the exact role of passive smoking in determining their appearance.

Important atherosclerotic changes are usually found in the arteries of old individuals who have not been exposed to passive smoking as a consequence of aging. Particularly, coronary and carotid arteries, those arterial locations where the negative effects of passive smoking exposure have been seen in any age, are affected by atherosclerotic changes in the elderly. Moreover, the alterations are almost similar in the two cases.

Cellular and molecular changes characterize the arteries of the elderly [39]. Artery wall elastic fibers are fragmented and reduced with an increase in collagen, so that the total content of elastin into the arterial wall is usually reduced by about one-third. Moreover, intima becomes thickened. With aging, deposits of lipids and calcium accumulate progressively into the media. It would seem that these processes, very similar to those of atherosclerosis, are age-related and may occur with or without concomitant development of an atherosclerotic plaque.

Finally, a concise comment needs to be made involving the behavior of systolic blood pressure in old patients, since this parameter increases as a consequence of the above mentioned changes in arterial structure but, at the same time, it influences structural changes. Isolated systolic hypertension, that is the most common form of hypertension over age 50, even when is mild in severity, usually is associated with a significant increase in cardiovascular disease risk [40–41]. Alterations sustained by isolated systolic hypertension could be worsened by exposure to passive smoking even if it is hard to establish the exact degree of impairment.

However, there are reports that underline the harmful effects of passive smoking exposure on cardiovascular system of the elderly individuals. Jaakkola [42] points out the potential role of environmental tobacco smoke exposure as a prognostic factor determining development of a pre-existing heart disease, going back to some of the epidemiological studies analyzed in Chapter 8. Analyzing, particularly, the studies of Steenland et al, Law et al, Thun et al, Donnan et al, Bonita et al, and Shinton and Beevers [13, 43 – 47], the author recognized that there was accumulating evidence suggesting that passive smoking exposure at home and in the workplace caused both coronary heart disease and stroke with a major incidence also in elderly individuals. The latter population, however, was included in those studies and moreover, the long follow-up led into old age some individuals who, when they had been enrolled into the study, were pre-senile subjects.

It is difficult, however, in these cases to identify those lesions which belong to passive smoking exposure or instead, to the elderly.

Cardiovascular changes that may affect elderly people, even after chronic exposure to passive smoking, should be evaluated prudentially and they would have less significance compared to those determined by other major coronary risk factors like combined systolic and diastolic blood pressure or diabetes mellitus [32].

References

[1] Westfall T, Cipolloni P, Edmundowicz A. Influence of propranolol on hemodynamic changes and plasma catecholamine levels following cigarette smoking and nicotine. *Proc. Soc. Exp. Biol. Med.* 1966; 123: 174 – 9.

[2] White S, McRitchie R. Nasopharingeal reflexes: integrative analysis of evoked respiratory and cardiovascular effects. *Aust. J. Exp. Biol. Med. Sci.* 1973; 51: 17 – 31.

[3] McMurray RG, Hicks LL, Thompson DL. The effects of passive inhalation of cigarette smoke on exercise performance. *Eur. J. Appl. Physiol.* 1985; 54: 196 – 200.

[4] Leone A. Il fumo di sigaretta: un potente fattore di rischio cardiovascolare. *Il Cuore.* 1991; 5: 573 – 80.

[5] Leone A, Bertanelli F, Mori L, Fabiano P, Battaglia A. Features of ischaemic cardiac pathology resulting from sigarette smoking. *J. Smoking-Related Dis.* 1994; 5: 109 – 14.

[6] Hole DJ, Gillis CR, Chopra C, Hawthorne VM. Passive smoking and cardiorespiratory health in a general population in the West of Scotland. *BMJ.* 1989; 299: 423 – 7.

[7] Glantz SA, Parmley WW. Passive smoking and heart disease : epidemiology, physiology, and biochemistry. *Circulation.* 1991; 83: 1 – 12.

[8] Leone A. Relationship between cigarette smoking and other coronary risk factors in atherosclerosis: risk of cardiovascular disease and preventive measures. *Curr. Pharm. Design.* 2003; 9: 2417 – 23.

[9] Barnoya J, Glantz SA. Cardiovascular effects of secondhand smoke. Nearly as large as smoking. *Circulation.* 2005; 111: 2684 – 98.

[10] Leone A, Lopez M. Oral contraception, ovarian disorders and tobacco in myocardial infarction of woman. *Pathologica.* 1986; 78: 237 – 42.

[11] Steenland K. Passive smoking and the risk of the heart disease. *JAMA.* 1992; 267: 94 – 9.

[12] Helsing K, Sandler D, Comstock G, Chee E. Heart disease mortality in nonsmokers living with smokers. *Am. J. Epidemiol.* 1988; 127: 915 – 22.

[13] Steenland K, Thun M, Lally C, Heath C Jr. Environmental tobacco smoke and coronary heart disease in the American Cancer Society CPS-II cohort. *Circulation.* 1996; 94: 622 – 8.

[14] Sandler DP, Comstock JW, Helsing KJ, Shore DL. Death from all causes in nonsmokers who lived with smokers. *Am. J. Public Health.* 1989; 79: 163 – 7.

[15] Svendsen KH, Kuller LK, Martin MJ, Ockene JF. Effects of passive smoking in the multiple risk factor intervention trials. *Am. J. Epidemiol.* 1987; 126: 783 – 95.

[16] He Y, Li L, Wang Z, Zheng X, Jia G. Women's passive smoking and coronary heart disease. *Chin. J. Prev. Med.* 1989; 23: 19 – 22.

[17] Humble C, Croft J, Gerber A, Casper M, Hames CG, Tyroler HA. Passive smoking and 20-year cardiovascular disease mortality among nonsmoking wives, Evans County, Georgia. *Am. J. Public Health.* 1990; 80: 599 – 601.

[18] He Y, Lam TH, Li LS, Du RY, Jia GL, Huang JY, Zheng JS. Passive smoking at work as a risk factor for coronary heart disease in Chinese women who have never smoked. *BMJ.* 1994; 308: 380 – 4.

[19] Layard MW. Ischemic heart disease and spousal smoking in the National Mortality Followback Survey. *Regular Toxicol. Pharmacol.* 1995; 21: 180 – 3.

[20] Matanoski G, Kanchanaraksa S, Lantry D, Chang J. Characteristics of nonsmoking women in NHANES I and NHANES I. Epidemiologic follow up study with exposure to spouses who smoke. *Am. J. Epidemiol.* 1995; 142; 149 – 57.

[21] Gilliland FD, Berhane K, McConnel R, Gauderman JW, Vora H, Rappaport EB, Avol E, Peters JM. Maternal smoking during pregnancy, environmental tobacco smoke exposure and childhood lung function. *Thorax.* 2000; 55: 271 – 6.

[22] Report of the California EPA (Environment Protection Agency), NCI (National Cancer Institute). Health effects of exposure to environmental tobacco smoke. 1999.

[23] Hawamdeh A, Kasasbeh FA, Ahmad MA. Effects of passive smoking on children's healths: a review. *Eastern Mediterranean Health Journal.* 2003; 9: 441 – 7.

[24] Malik S, Cleves M, Zhao W, Hobbs C. Congenital heart disease and maternal smoking. *Circulation.* 2006; 114 (18): 3274S.

[25] Kotulak R. Mom smoking, heart defect linked. *Chicago Tribune.* 2006, 11, 25.

[26] Rubin DH, Damus C. The relationship between passive smoking and child health: methodologic criteria applied to prior studies. *Yale J. Biol. Med.* 1988; 61: 401 – 11.

[27] Bakoula CG, Kafritsa YJ, Kavadias GD, Lazopoulou DD, Theodoridou MC, Maravelias KP, Matsaniotis NS. Objective passive-smoking indicators and respiratory morbidity in young children. *Lancet.* 1995; 346: 280 – 1.

[28] Shima M, Adachi M. Effects of environmental tobacco smoke on serum levels of acute phase proteins in schoolchildren. *Preventive Medicine.* 1996; 25: 617 – 24.

[29] Rossier ML, Fernandez Vega M, Villalba Caloca J, Letama CM, Flores Sanchez S. Frequency of acute respiratory infections in children of parents who smoke and children of nonsmoking parents. In *Tobacco and Health,* Slama K ed, Plenum Press, New York, 1995; 537 – 9.

[30] Weisfeldt ML. Aging of the cardiovascular system. *N. Engl. J. Med.* 1980; 303; 1172 - 4.

[31] Kannel WB, Gordon T. Evaluation of cardiovascular risk in the elderly: The Framingham Study. *Bull. NY Acad. Med.* 1978; 54: 573 – 91.

[32] Bertoncini G, Bertanelli F, Leone A. Coronary risk factors (CRF) in acute myocardial infarction (AMI) of elderly with and without hypertension. *AJ. H.* 1999; 12: 197 A, 002.

[33] Davies HEF. Respiratory change in heart rate, sinus arrhythmia in the elderly. *Gerontol. Clin.* 1975; 17: 96 - 100.

[34] Gribbin B, Pickering TG, Sleight P, Peto R. Effect of age and high blood pressure on baroreflex sensitivity in man. *Circ. Res.* 1971; 29: 424 – 31.

[35] Rothbaum DA, Shaw DJ, Angell CS, Shock NW. Cardiac performance in the unanesthetized senescent male rat. *J. Gerontol.* 1973; 28: 287 – 292.

[36] Ritch AES. The significance of carotid sinus hypersensitivity in the elderly. *Gerontol. Clin.* 1975; 17: 146 – 53.

[37] Smiddy J, Lewis HD Jr, Dunn M. The effect of carotid massage in older men. *J. Gerontol.* 1972; 27: 209 – 11.

[38] Vestal RE, Wood AJJ, Shand DG. Reduced Beta-adrenoreceptor sensitivity in the elderly. *Clin. Pharmacol. Ther.* 1979; 26: 181 – 6.

[39] Lakatta EG. Cellular and molecular clues to heart and arterial aging. *Circulation.* 2003; 107: 490 – 7.

[40] Franklin SS, Larson MG, Khan SA, Wong ND, Leip EP, Kannel WB, Levy D. Does the relation of blood pressure to coronary heart disease risk change with aging? The Framingham Heart Study. *Circulation.* 2001; 103: 1245 – 9.

[41] Sesso HD, Stampfer MJ, Rosner B, Hennekens CH, Gaziano MJ, Manson JAE, Glynn RJ. Systolic and diastolic blood pressure, pulse pressure, and mean arterial pressure as predictors of cardiovascular disease risk in men. *Hypertension.* 2000; 36: 801 – 7.

[42] Jaakkola MS. Environmental tobacco smoke and health in the elderly. *Eur. Respir. J.* 2002; 19: 172 – 81.

[43] Law MR, Morris JK, Wald NJ. Environmental tobacco smoke exposure and ischaemic heart disease: an evaluation of the evidence. *BMJ.* 1997; 315: 973 – 80.

[44] Thun M, Henley J, Apicella L. Epidemiologic studies on fatal and nonfatal cardiovascular disease and ETS exposure from spousal smoking. *EHP.* 1999, 107 (Suppl 6) : 841 – 6.

[45] Donnan GA, McNeil JJ, Adena MA, Doyle AE, O'Malley HM, Neill GC. Smoking as a risk factor for cerebral ischaemia. *Lancet.* 1989; 2: 643 – 7.

[46] Bonita R, Duncan J, Truelsen T, Jackson RT, Beaglehole R. Passive smoking as well as active smoking increases the risk of acute stroke. *Tobacco Control.* 1999; 8: 156 – 60.

[47] Shinton R, Beevers G. Meta-analysis of relation between cigarette smoking and stroke. *BMJ.* 1989; 298: 789 – 94.

Chapter 11

FROM A RISK TO AN ETIOLOGIC FACTOR: HOW TO BUILD A MATHEMATICAL MODEL

ABSTRACT

There are a lot of study approaches: clinical, biological, metabolic, epidemiologic, statistic and so on, that recognize different pathogenetic mechanisms of damage. Nowadays, there is no doubt that exposure to passive smoking, whenever it may be approached to be studied, and leads to only one final result that is a reversibly functional harm of the heart and blood vessels following acute exposure, and pathologic alterations that become, in the long run, irreversible lesions of the above target organs after chronic exposure.

The degree of cardiovascular damage caused by passive smoking exposure depends on three factors- type of smoking, environment, and study subject - as well as by numerous variables which may be related to them. Possibly quantifying the numerous variables related to smoking, environment, and individuals, permit one to build a mathematical equation that establishes the level of damage as well as its exact reproducibility, as observed for a single subject in one study.

Since passive smoking exposure leads undoubtedly, in the long run, to cardiovascular pathology, this factor must be considered an etiologic factor, namely a factor with a bind cause-effect, of cardiovascular disease.

Keywords: Risk factor, etiologic factor, mathematical model, result(s) reproducibility, passive smoking exposure, cardiovascular system.

Assessing the exact role that passive smoking exposure has in determining cardiovascular damage is of a basic importance since, as said previously, different opinions exist on the subject.

These different opinions are based on the fact that several reports often reach different results either on the type and degree of damage induced or on its relationship with passive smoking exposure. Therefore, there is demand to unanimously interpret the significance and role of passive smoking exposure to give a correct setting to cardiovascular damage. Indeed, establishing well what is due to passive smoking and what is due to different factors in inducing the damage is hard but nowadays, possiblly analyzing the findings on the relationship between the two factors. Findings conclude, almost similarly, that passive smoking exposure is a major risk factor for cardiovascular system.

In my opinion, the above statement is limiting for the effective role developed by passive smoking. A critical question arises: is passive smoking exposure only a major cardiovascular risk factor or, on the contrary, it reveals characteristics of major importance in the light of the results obtained by the researches on the subject .

Really, the two most important factors enable one to interpret the probable incidence of appearance for every disease. They have a strongly epidemiological significance since their identification permits to assess clinical, therapeutical and prognostic approach to the disease itself. These factors are known respectively as risk factors, that is, today, they are carefully considered to assess the incidence of a disease and then set up preventive measures, and etiologic factor, which is the specific cause of a disease, the occurence of which is the close result of the strength and potential charge of this factor.

Trying to establish the potential approaches to these factors when one interprets the results derived by findings on passive smoking exposure permits to specify, carefully, the role of passive smoking on cardiovascular system.

A risk factor is a variable usually associated with the appearance of disease with a major incidence although it does not necessarily play a causal role. For example, when one analyzes if coronary heart disease recognizes some variables which can cause it, there is evidence of the absence of a specific factor capable always cause the disease, but there will be several events like hypertension, high cholesterol level, diabetes mellitus, and so on that, with elevated but different rate, may accompany alone or all together the appearance of the disease. Therefore, one can conclude that there are factors that may help the appearance of a disease although they do not necessarily determine the appearance.

The power of a risk factor may be asssessed by comparing the risk of those subjects exposed to the specific factor who show an event to those without it by a ratio that is as follows:

Number of Subjects Experiencing an Event in Presence of a Known Factor

Total Number of Subjects

Statistical methods are capable to establish the level and power of a risk factor by comparing the percent of population affected negatively by its presence on the total population. As there is evidence, it is really impossible to analyze the whole population and therefore, a degree of different probability will characterize such an estimate, as well as it has been described in the chapter treating the statistical methodologies to be applied.

A risk factor provides the global burden of disease by the analysis of a lot of events which involve lifestyle, age and gender, socioeconomic states, education, geagraphical area characteristics and other characteristics of the studied population. Assessing, possibly, the maximum number of parameters related to a specific risk factor is useful to establish its potential effect in a better way.

Risk factors can be divided into two categories: 1. Risk factors strongly related to increased incidence of a disease. Two occurences may characterize this statement: the removal of the risk factor can induce a real decrease in incidence of the disease or, on the contrary, the risk factor cannot be removed and therefore, no decrease in incidence of the disease may be seen. Therefore, further studies need to change the latter pattern; 2. Risk factors that might be related to increased incidence of a disease. Here also, there exist two possibilities: the first is that of risk factor removal with possible decrease in incidence of the disease thus, further studies would need to clarify how risk factor may be removed or its effects reduced; the second way recognizes a risk factors which is unable to be removed. On this occurence, no decrease in incidence of the disease may be identified and therefore, no further study needs to be conducted to interpret the relationship between risk factor and examined disease. Table 11.1. lists the main cardiovascular risk factors classified according to the aforesaid statements.

Table 11.1. Main cardiovascular risk factors classified according to their characteristics

Characteristic	Risk factor	Removal/reduction
1. Risk factor strongly related to a heart disease	LDL-Cholesterol	Possible
	Hypertension	Possible
	Smoking	Possible
	Diabetes mellitus	possible
	Aging	No possible
	Obesity	possible
	Metabolic syndrome	possible
2. Risk factor probably related to heart disease	Familial history	No possible
	No physical activity	possible
	Recurrent stress	possible
	Inflammation	possible
	Homocysteine	possible

As one can see, among the factors strongly related to a cardiovascular disease, there are all the major cardiovascular risk factors which, moreover, could be removed or reduced in power by preventive measures or pharmacological therapy. Smoking, particularly, may act as a factor capable to cause cardiovascular damage as well as a factor that potentiates the effects of the others. However, it would be a risk factor which is possible to avoid, even if with evident difficulties.

The results provided by the exam of the risk factors are usually deriving from epidemiological studies. The larger the epidemiological study, the better the risk factor may be interpreted. However, there is no link of cause-effect between a risk factor and occurence of disease. On the contrary, it has the strongest links with its own etiologic factor, as it will be discussed ahead.

Analysis of risk factors for passive smoking permitted establish that the risk of death from cardiovascular disease rise by up to 30 percent among those individuals who are chronically exposed to environmental tobacco smoke at home or in workplaces [2]. It is also estimated that about 35,000 non smokers die from cardiovascular events each year as a consequence of passive smoking exposure [3].

Therefore, it is important to know how a risk factor acts on a particular disease in a large series of findings as well as in a large number of subjects with different geographical origin and lifestyle. It is necessary to estimate the possibility to remove the risk factors, particularly when it plays a strong role, in significatively reducing the incidence of a disease as well as intercurrent related events, making any effort to obtain that.

An emerging concept to prevent the incidence of cardiovascular disease is to carry out those strategies to prevent the negative effects of risk factors [4]. Indeed, smoking is a risk factor that could be completely removed even if with a great effort. However, exposure to passive smoking should be avoided if this factor is believed to be only a risk factor, but absolutely legally forbidden if a leading role as a causal factor of cardiovascular damage can be demonstrated. In my opinion, the latter statement is true in the light of results obtained by several findings and therefore establishing what is an etiologic factor, basic to interpret correctly the negative effects of passive smoking exposure on cardiovascular system.

The concept that some abnormal symptoms or diseases recognize a causal factor, namely etiologic factor, is as ancient as medical history [5]. In more modern terms, there are two major classes of etiologic factors: genetic and acquired etiologic factors. They bind the disease that cause by a relation of cause-effect. However, the appearance of the disease, clinically evident, derives from the power inherent from the causal factor. Level, power, and duration of the etiologic factors determine different patterns of illness severity.

The purpose of identifying an etiologic factor for the largest number of diseases is the effort of contemporary findings since its knowledge permits a careful approach to disease diagnosis, treatment, but also a prognostic estimate of the damage caused. The latter parameter is what is interesting in passive smoking findings since to establish exactly the type and progression of a damage is basic to carry out those strategies capable to avoid or reduce its negative effects.

Therefore, analyzing if passive smoking exposure has a bind cause-effect and then may be considered an etiologic factor of cardiovascular disease is undoubtedly useful to clarify the harm produced by environmental tobacco smoke. By the knowledge of the concept of mathematical models, one can reach a clear answer to the above concept.

BUILDING A MATHEMATICAL MODEL

Considerable progresses have been made over the last decade in developing, validating, and testing mathematical models to predict the response of a system to known factors and therefore identify the main functional and structural characteristic of the system.

Firstly used in physics and engineering, mathematical models tend to spread out different fields of biological and medical sciences, particularly for what is concerning environment characteristics as well as establishing therapeutic protocols or possible plasma concentrations of metabolites. All mathematical models use an equation where two expressions indicated by the sign = (equal) take part to calculate the numerical value of an unknown term. A careful estimate for predicting indoor air quality by using a mathematical model has been published recently by Ott [6]. For passive smoking, the concentrations of pollutants depend on different factors related to the environment, number of cigarettes smoked into, number of persons and exponential decay once the cigarette ends. For what is concerning exposed individuals, a mathematical model, to be effective, must quantify and reproduce an experimental finding. Indeed, only a reproducibility of a study confirms its validation as well as objectify obtained results.

Therefore, a critical question that arises is: can we build a mathematical model to assess cardiovascular damage from passive smoking exposure as well as its reproducibility, and if yes, how?

In a previous chapter (chapter 7), one could observe that statistical and epidemiological studies analyzed individuals who were different from themselves particularly for a lot of habits, although the great number of subjects included into the study samples led to the conclusion, validated statistically, that cardiovascular damage from passive smoking exposure existed, in spite of a different degree of statistical significance. This statement was the result of the fact that epidemiological studies on passive smoking exposure exceeded one of the limits of statistical methods, particularly the small number of studied individuals since, usually, they were large-scale studies. However, recording too much information as a purpose of statistical studies on large-scale, even if favorable for a percent estimate of a damage, could lead to confusion [7] in evaluating obtained results with care, as believed by experts in statistics, because of the unsimilar applying of study protocol, particularly when findings were multicenter trials .

A previous finding that validates a mathematical model to be built, since it gave exactly reproducible results, although derived from a single subject, is that published by Leone [8]. This experimental human finding has got what is required for building a mathematical model: steady measures of passive smoking component concentrations during exercise performed in passive smoking exposure, same characteristics of the studied subject, equal type of exposure. So, one could build a mathematical equation using similar parameters.

Briefly, in 1989 a 58-year-old man first presented with an aterior myocardial infarction at the Coronary Care Unit of the Hospital. Six months later, coronary angiography showed that the left anterior descending artery was totally occluded. Patient refused cardiac surgery for arterial revascularization. However, serial exercise testings performed according to the method of Fletcher and Schlant [9] did not show ischemic and/or arrhythmic alterations. Furthermore, the patient was asymptomatic when beta-blocker therapy (propranolol 120 mg/daily) was administered. Five years later, the patient gave his informed consent to undergo a study into the effects of passive smoking according to a modification of a method of Leone et al. [10]. He underwent 4 sessions of exercise stress testing on a bicycle ergometer, during which he was exposed alternatively to a smoke-free environment and an environment polluted with 30 to 35 parts per million air carbon monoxide concentration derived from burned tobacco. Plasma carboxyhemoglobin concentration measured before and after exercise was similar for the two pre-exposure and increased similarly during the two post-exposure to passive smoking. Electrocardiogram recordings during both sessions in the smoke-free environment showed a mild sinus tachycardia. During the two exercises in the polluted environment, similar and quantitatively, the same bigeminal ventricular ectopic beats occurred which necessitated the stopping of exercise. Therefore, this post-myocardial infarction patient showed exactly reproducible life-threatening ventricular arrhythmias when exercising in a same smoke-environment polluted by carbon monoxide in a concentration usually found in public places where active smokers stay.

Therefore, when one approaches an experiment on the relationship between passive smoking exposure and cardiovascular response with almost similar procedures, obtained results are always the same.

Possibly, all those variables that may be related with an experiment should be adjusted to the environment, type of exposure, and exposed subject when the results following environmental tobacco smoke are analyzed.

Building a mathematical equation of exposure to passive smoking needs to consider three main parameters with their variables, that usually are a large number. Some variables are related to passive smoking concentrations, some to the characteristics of the environment, and some more to the exposed subjects. Parameters like duration and type of exposure, chemical concentrations in the environment, cubic content of the environment, age and sex of the exposed subject as well as his socio-economic and health status, and so on, must be standardized when an experimental finding is conducted.

However, indicating the variables by the letters a, b, c as well as n equal to the number of possible factors of each variable, the mathematical equation to quantify exactly cardiovascular damage from passive smoking (P value) is as follows:

$$\frac{(na + nb + nc)}{n\,(abc)}$$

For a P value, that analyzes all the possibilities of mathematical combination, equal to 1.

As one can deduce from the knowledge of what has been described about the significance of the statistical certainty (see also Chapter 7), a number equal to 1 is expression of a 100% of validation.

Cardiovascular damage from passive smoking may be assessed quantitatively by using a mathematical model that requires exactly similar experimental procedures. When such a condition exist, the reproducibility of the results characterizes each single experiment.

Therefore, by the analysis of different reports as well as by building a mathematical model, passive smoking has to be considered an etiologic factor, namely a factor characterized by a bind cause-effect, of cardiovascular disease since it leads, in the long run, to the evident developing of cardiovascular pathology, although different levels of damage due to a numerous factors related to the main three variables, environment, smoking exposure and exposed subject, may be observed and then, must be carefully quantified. Moreover, passive smoking exposure could be easily avoided, canceling its negative effects, if strong efforts towards this measure are conducted.

References

[1] Leone A. Passive smoking exposure and cardiovascular health. In: *Passive Smoking and Health Research,* Jeorgensen NA ed, Nova Science Publishers, Inc. 2006 (in press).

[2] He J, Vupputury S, Allen K, Prerost MR, Hughes J, Whelton PK. Passive smoking and the risk of coronary heart disease- A meta-analysis of epidemiologic studies. *N. Engl. J. Med.* 1999; 340: 920 – 6.

[3] World Health Organization. The World Health Report 2002: *Reducing risks, promoting healthy life*. Geneva 2002: WHO.

[4] Benjamin EJ, Smith SC Jr, Cooper RS, Hill MN, Luepker RV. Task Force # 1- magnitude of the prevention problem: Opportunities and challanges. 33rd Bethesda Conference. *J. Am. Coll. Cardiol.* 2002; 40: 588 – 603.

[5] Majno G. The Healing Hand. Cambridge, MA, Harward University Press, 1975: 43.

[6] Ott WR. Mathematical models for predicting indoor air quality. *Environ Health Perspect.* 1999; 107: 375 – 81.

[7] Wright P, Haybittle J. Design of forms for clinical trials. *BMJ.* 1979; ii: 650 – 1.

[8] Leone A. Passive smoking causes cardiac alterations in post-MI subjects. *Int. J. Smoking Cessation.* 1996; 3: 42 – 3.

[9] Fletcher GF, Schlant RC. The exercise test. In: Hurst's the Heart, 8th Ed, Schlant RC and Alexander WR eds. McGraw-Hill, New York 1994; 423 – 40.

[10] Leone A, Mori L, Bertanelli F, Fabiano P, Filippelli M. Indoor passive smoking: its effect on cardiac performance. *Int. J. Cardiol.* 1991; 8: 247 – 52.

Chapter 12

PREVENTIVE MEASURES AGAINST DAMAGE: CLEAN AIR

ABSTRACT

Passive smoking, an etiologic factor for cardiovascular disease, must be fought by using all those measures capable to avoid or reduce its negative effects similarly to what is usually made against etiologic factors of the other diseases.

To obtain that, it is necessary to know and change the interaction among different major cardiovascular risk factors that have been demonstrated capable to potentiate passive smoking effects.

Association of passive smoking particularly with elevated concentrations of LDL-cholesterol and/or hypertension potentiates harmful effects exponentially of more than three or four times than those passive smoking alone. Young people are affected mainly when this association occurs. However, negative effects in every phase of life have been demonstrated.

Preventive measures to reduce passive smoking effects must be addressed to the individuals by using diet supplementation, physical activity, and sometimes, pharmacological interventions, as well as the environment to obtain cleaner air because of a reduction of smoke pollutants.

Since data confirm that architectural characteristics of the different buildings permit one to live in healthy environments, efforts must be made to reduce outdoor and indoor air pollution due to smoking of active smokers.

Keywords: Prevention, Risk factor(s) interaction, passive smoking, LDL-cholesterol, hypertension, clean air, policy issue, sick building syndrome.

Negative effects of passive smoking exposure on cardiovascular system have been widely described in the previous chapters. One can unbiasedly conclude that environmental tobacco smoke is an etiologic rather than a risk factor of cardiovascular disease.

Therefore, exposure must be fought by using all those measures capable to avoid or reduce, in a more possible way, its negative effects similarly to what is usually made against etiologic factors of the other diseases. As an example, the use of antibiotics eradicates some infective diseases and therapeutic effects of these drugs are utilized whenever it needs. Similarly, passive smoking exposure could be legally forbidden and, by this way, canceled its harmful effects. However, even if easy to say, it is very difficult to realize. Thus, all those measures that can reduce the harm must be carefully analyzed to reach reduced negative effects of smoking exposure. Primarily, for what concern cardiovascular system since negative effects of passive smoking lead to the appearance of atherosclerosis, coronary heart disease and stroke, the relationship between passive smoking and other major coronary risk factors should be well interpreted to avoid, at least, their synergistic effects.

Relationship between Passive Smoking and other Major Risk Factors

Interesting observations on the possible interaction of cardiovascular risk factors derive from the results provided by different studies of which MRFIT cohort large-study [1] is of a particular significance.

From the analysis of this study, it emerges that everyone of the major coronary risk factors, namely cholesterol level, hypertension, smoking and diabetes mellitus, isolatedly exerts a strong effect in increasing the rate of appearance of coronary events for those people who show the risk factor. Moreover, when these major factors are combined among them, their effects increase exponentially and the increase may be also measured [2 – 3]. For example, if hypothetically a risk factor alone increases the risk of appearance of a cardiovascular event by 10 %, its power is raised by 4 to 5 times when other coronary risk factors are associated in different combinations among them. Such a fact leads to an increase per cent, when interaction between major risk factors occurs, up to 70 to 80% compared to the effects of a single risk factor. However, some differences according to the type of associated factors exist. Usually, strongly potentiated effects demonstrate the association between level of LDL-cholesterol, smoking and hypertension in young people, whereas diabetes mellitus, isolated systolic hypertension and both systolic and diastolic hypertension associated play a heavy effect in elderly subjects. However, the degree of risk is absolutely increased when these conditions occur.

Smoking well relates its negative effects on cardiovascular system particularly with LDL-Cholesterol concentrations since both factors are capable to induce, in time, atherosclerotic plaque formation. Passive smoking too potentiates its negative effects when high LDL-Choleterol levels are associated.

A study assessing the interaction among the major coronary risk factors [4] analyzed the association of cholesterol, triglycerides, blood pressure, obesity, and cigarette smoking. Two methods were used: standard correlation analysis, and percentile analysis method applying of which was limited to associations at higher levels of these risk factors. Percentile analysis requires that known values of a variable are divided into 100 sub-sets with equal frequencies. Mathematical result of a percentile is easy to be calculated, being the ratio of the number of observations below the value to be analyzed, divided the total number of observations multiplied by 100. The study population consisted of 4,839 men and women aged from 30 to 39 years, a number statistically significant. In the percentile analysis, subjects with moderate or greater (equal or over 70th percentile) or high (equal or over 90th percentile) levels on one of the examined risk factors showed clustering of elevations in other risk factors in that expected ratios were generally greater than unity, excepting smoking comparisons. However, from these data there is a clear incidence of the strongest power due to interactions of the major coronary risk factors.

Data provided by the report of Gotto [3] pointed out that the mortality rate from coronary heart disease was from two to three times greater in those people who were heavy smokers, representing smoking as an independent major risk factor for coronary heart disease. Moreover, the risk was even higher when smokers were also hypertensive and with elevated levels of cholesterol, a pathological status of a frequent observation in ischemic patients.

Interaction between smoking and other major coronary risk factors has also been analyzed by other papers [5–9].

Pooling Project [7] provides further data about risk factors interaction. A synergic effect of cigarette smoking with hypertension and elevated cholesterol levels was also demonstrated. Moreover, in the Ni-Hon-San Study [8] the effects of cigarette smoking on ischemic heart disease rate in the presence of hypercholesterolemia appeared to be more than additive in the Japanese Americans who lived in Hawaii. The same effect, however, was not observed in Japanese men living in Japan, who usually have lower cholesterol levels. Furtherly, there was a synergic effect [9] among the different major coronary risk factors also in the Goteborg study.

The interaction among all the major coronary risk factors, although clearly identified, does not fully explain the greater response of some population genetically protected. Synergism, however, could explain the different cardiovascular disease rate in those people having a genetic protection when they are compared to those who have no such state.

Multiple logistic equations have been prepared and applied to establish the level of interaction of the major coronary risk factors. These equations analyze the presence of multiple risk factors with additive effects within themselves. Indeed, when one estimates the degree of the intaraction adding the percent value of each factor, the obtained result is lower that that represented by real value of the risk due to the association. Such a condition is clearly explained by the fact that not a mathematical addition, but an exponential increase regulates the power of coronary risk factors when they are acting together.

Analytical and methodological refinements appear to be useful for a better knowledge of coronary risk factor synergism. Nevertheless, the evidence exists that cigarette smoking greatly increases the risk of cardiovascular events in individuals already at increased risk because of other risk factor presence.

Since the power of smoking as a risk factor depends on, as already described, the concentrations of its toxic compounds, the same constituents in either active smoking or passive smoking, the different amounts in toxic chemicals (usually higher in active smoking). They could influence the type of response to passive smoking exposure at a lower level when it is associated with other major cardiovascular risk factors. Anyway, this is a superfluous statement since, as already described, passive smoking exposure should be considered as an etiologic factor of cardiovascular disease. Therefore, even if interaction between passive smoking and other coronary risk factors occurs at a level lower than that of active smoking, there is no doubt that the association with the other risk factors potentiates the negative effects of passive smoking on the cardiovascular system.

Finally, it is good to keep in mind that no individual risk factor is essential or sufficient in the onset of cardiovascular events. Usually, a multifactorial etiology may be recognized for cardiovascular disease. Thus, multivariate risk factor assessment provides useful measures of the joint level by risk factor alone or combined with others. Therefore, multivariate analysis of coronary risk factors permit to give effective guidelines for preventing a disease. For what is concerning the type of cardiovascular event that may occur in individuals with multiple risk factors, there is no explanation on the fact that a cardiovascular event may be fatal or nonfatal with regards to a possibly different association of risk factors, being the appearance of a negative event under control of a lot of other factors, the knowledge of which is yet to be interpreted. Therefore, when we are in presence of association among different major risk factors, a global burden of their effects may be, statistically, measured but no information can be obtained on the outcome of disease.

PREVENTIVE MEASURES: CLEAN AIR

The main preventive measures to carry out for what concerns a reduction of individuals' disorders due to passive smoking exposure at a metabolic, functional, dietary and physical level have been described in Chapter 6, where the role of oxidative stress was analyzed. Briefly, diet supplementation, physical activity and sometimes pharmacological approaches might be followed to improve the health of those subjects who had been chronically exposed to passive smoking, often associated with other risk factors. Moreover, the role of the main characteristics of an environment have also been analyzed in Chapter 1, since the environment itself must be considered, sometimes, a risk factor.

Here, the more effective measures to build an environment that may protect individuals from the negative effects of passive smoking will be briefly described in the light of what has been assessed until now for those cardiovascular parameters particularly changed by the exposure.

An individual living in both outdoor and indoor environments breathes usually from 3 to 9 litres of air per minute. Moreover, it is known that the environment is polluted by a lot of chemicals from industries as well as car traffic that cause an air pollution estimated, only for the latter parameter, equal to more than 50 percent. Therefore, individuals pay a heavy tribute to the major pollutants of the modern society.

Aspecific symptoms related to poor indoor air quality in several nonindustrial buildings have been reported [10] and described with the term of sick building syndrome. Symptoms described are common in the general population and may be influenced by a large variety of factors. Sick building syndrome was related to many air pollutants and, for what concerned passive smoking, the exposure mainly affected those children who had been exposed to maternal tobacco smoke. On the contrary, little or no effect was associated with residential factors such of age and type of building, degree of crowding, mechanical ventilation, moisture or mold growth. Therefore, architectural elements did not damage living people who could have different breathing troubles as a consequence of chemical, biological and allergenic air pollutants. Thus, preventive measures must be addressed to clean air into the different environments.

In recent years [11–13], the role of the environment in influencing individual smoking behavior has been increasingly recognized. In many indoor environments, that have been carefully monitored to assess smoking pollutants, environmental tobacco smoke has been detected.

Findings consistently show that the concentrations of a number of toxic constituents from burned cigarettes were elevated in those environments where smoking was allowed, as compared to those where it was not. Moreover, as already described, data [14–17] would demonstrate that reached value of smoke components are as high to be dosed in biological fluids of nonsmoker exposed individuals. A further concept to be considered is that passive smoking constituents may also aggregate with other pollutant components in the air and, by doing so, may change in character and, moreover, potentiate their effects. Notwithstanding that, health risks related to smokeless tobacco have received comparatively little attention, in spite of widespread use in many parts of the world [18].

To have absolutely clean air, an analysis of what may be changed is basic to be conducted. Since the pollutants from industries and car traffic are unmodifiable components of individuals' lifestyle, there is a need to remove or reduce all those additional chemicals that can pollute the air. In this way, passive smoking exposure could be reduced significantly.

Environmental and policy interventions would be among the most cost-effective approaches to reach in an attempt to obtain a reduced degree of passive smoking exposure. One of the most useful ways is by adopting clean air policies everywhere.

Indeed, several legal acts are more and more arising to fight passive smoking air pollution. In this way, the United States are advancing quickly [19]. Some local health departments have been authorized to bring about reforms of clean air defence, forbidding to smoke in public buildings. Also tobacco advertising has been banned in several countries, although it financed a lot of cultural and sport events which did not have any financial support [21]. Table 12.1. summarizes the main legal issues promoted as well as those to be added to obtain clean air from tobacco smoke. As one can see, a large majority of these measures are policy interventions that are the main guidelines to obtain a control of smoking habit and, consequently, reduce pollution due to passive smoking exposure.

Table 12.1. Mean policy issues promoted and issues to be added for tobacco control

Issues promoted	Law designs
	Restricting advertising
	Educational programs
	Increased price of cigarettes
Issues to be added	Insurance differential premium
	Incentives for stopping smoking
	Promoting individual fitness
	Regular lessons to schoolboys
	Control of tobacco production
	Unifying law worldwide

By applying together all these measures, it might be hypothesized that clean air from tobacco exposure is feasible with a significant reduction of the harm represented by passive smoking that affects negatively all the phases of life, and of which cardiovascular system is a target organ.

References

[1] Stamler J, Wentworth D, Neaton JD, for the MRFIT Cooperative Research Group. Is the relationship between serum cholesterol and risk of death from coronary heart disease continuous and graded ? Findings on 356,222 primary screenees of the Multiple Risk Factor Intervention Trial (MRFIT). *JAMA.* 1986; 256: 2823 – 8.

[2] Cornfield J. Joint dependence of risk of coronary heart disease on serum cholesterol and systolic blood pressure: A discriminant function and analysis. *Fed. Proc.* 1962; 21 (Suppl II): 58 – 61.

[3] Gotto AM Jr. Interactions of the major risk factors for coronary heart disease. *Am. J. Med.* 1986; 80 (Suppl 2A): 48 – 55.

[4] Criqui MH, Barret-Connor E, Holdbrook MJ, Austin M, Turner JD. Clustering of cardiovascular disease risk factors. *Preventive Medicine.* 1980; 9: 525 – 33.

[5] Carlson LA, Bottiger LE, Ahfeldt PE. Risk factors for myocardial infarction in the Stockholm Prospective Study. A 14-year follow-up focussing on the role of plasma triglycerides and cholesterol. *Acta Medica Scandinavica.* 1979; 206: 351 – 60.

[6] Kannel WB. Some lessons in cardiovascular epidemiology from Framingham. *Am. J. Cardiol.* 1976: 37: 269 – 82.

[7] Pooling Project Research Group. Relationship of blood pressure, serum cholesterol, smoking habit, relative weight and ECG abnormalities to incidence of major coronary event: Final report of the Pooling Project. *J. Chronic Dis.* 1978: 31: 201 – 306.

[8] Robertson TL, Kato H, Gordon T, Kagan A, Rhoads GG, Land CE, Worth RM, Belsky JL, Dock DS, Miyanishi M, Kawamoto S. Epidemiologic studies of coronary heart disease and stroke in Japanese men living in Japan, Hawaii and California. Coronary heart disease risk factors in Japan and Hawaii. *Am. J. Cardiol.* 1977; 39: 244 –9.

[9] Wilhelmsen L. Risk factors for disease according to population studies in Goteborg, Sweden. In: *Medical Aspects of Mortality Statistics.* Skandinavia International Symposia, Bostrom H and Ljungstedt N eds, Almquist and Wiksell International, Stockholm 1981; 73 – 88.

[10] Norback D, Edling C. Environmental, occupational, and personal factors related to the prevalence of sick building syndrome in the general population. *Br. J. Ind. Med.* 1991; 48: 451 – 62.

[11] National Cancer Institute: Strategies to control tobacco use in the United States: A blueprint for public health action in the 1990s. Smoking and Tobacco Control Monographs 1. Bethesda, MD, National Cancer Institute, U.S. Department of Health and Human Services, 1991 (NIH Pub. No. 92-3316).

[12] McKinlay JB. The promotion of health through planned sociopolitical change: Challenges for research and policy. *Soc. Sci. Med.* 1993; 36: 109 – 17.

[13] Brownson RC, Matson Koffman D, Novotny TE, Hughes RG, Eriksen MP. Environmental and policy interventions to control tobacco use and prevent cardiovascular disease. *Health Education Quarterly.* 1995; 22: 478 – 98.

[14] Benowitz NL. Cotinine as a biomarker of environmental tobacco smoke exposure. *Epidemiol. Rev.* 1996; 18: 188 – 204.

[15] Benowitz NL, Jacob P. Nicotine and cotinine elimination pharmacokinetics in smokers and non smokers. *Clin. Pharmacol. Ter.* 1993; 53: 316 – 23.

[16] Vogt TM, Selvin S, Widdowson G, Hulley SB. Expired air carbon monoxide and serum thiocyanate as objective measures of cigarette exposure. *Am. J. Public Health.* 1977; 67: 545 – 9.

[17] Ekemin SA, Coxon RE, Colbert DL, Landon J, Smith DS. Urinary cotinine fluoroimmunoassay for smoking status screening adapted to an automated analyser. *Analyst.* 1992; 117: 697 – 9.

[18] Pershagen G. Smokeless tobacco. *British Medical Bulletin.* 1996; 52: 50 – 7.

[19] Rigotti NA, Pashos CL. No-smoking laws in the United States. An analysis of state and city action to limit smoking in public places and workplaces. *JAMA.* 1991; 266: 3162 – 7.

[20] Coalition on Smoking or Health. State legislated actions on tobacco issues. Washington, DC, 1993.

[21] Laws MB, Whitman J, Bowser DM, Krech L. Tobacco availability and point of sale marketing in demographically contrasing districts of Massachusets. *Tobacco Control.* 2002; 11: 71 – 3.

Chapter 13

FINAL REMARKS

From the wide mosaic of papers analyzed for assessing the effects of passive smoking exposure on heart and blood vessels, the most important of which have been reported as references in chapters of this book, these reports focus on those elements related to the specific subject which was treated, some interesting data need to be memorized to correctly interpret cardiovascular damage as a "photograph".

The first concept to remove is the distortion of the thought in assessing the relationship between harmful effects of passive smoking exposure and cardiovascular system: believing or not that passive smoking exposure is a negative occurence. One must have certain data about existing damage, and not just believe.

From the book opening to its end, these statements must be kept in mind to reach such a demonstration.

1. The particular shape of tobacco leaves associated with soil moisture permit to clarify important characteristics which need to be considered to go into details of the acting mechanism concerning passive smoking. The shape of the leaf like a "cupule" permits an uniform distribution of its alkaloids of which nicotine is particularly soluble in water and then, a maximum amount of extraction occurs. Nicotine is one the most toxic components, not only of passive smoking, but also acting as fresh leaves. One must keep in mind that this step does not involve carbon monoxide that originates during cigarette burning.
2. Nicotine burns at a temperature of 240°C that is below its boiling point (247°C). Chemically, that means that nicotine is burned particularly when a cigarette is still smoked. Smoker then inhales the alkaloid, and alkaloid also diffuses into the environment before its decomposition. Therefore, nicotine may almost entirely play its adverse effects. Although nicotine has the peculiar property of autoignition before its boiling point, a lower amount than the total of the tobacco leaf is dosable in the different types of smoke. Also carbon monoxide, considered the most toxic component of environmental tobacco smoke, begins to arouse its effects during this phase.
3. Characteristics of the environment. The level of some smoke constituents in the environmental tobacco smoke depends closely on the environment space, ventilation rate, decay rate, mixing rate, and room volume as well as number of cigarette

smoked into the environment, number of nonsmoker people present and current presence or absence of active smokers. Since it is well known that architectural structure of modern buildings permits indoor healthy life, the pollutants which are present in the air, both indoor and outdoor air, cause damage to health. Passive smoking toxics spread out and also aggregate other air pollutants and, by doing so, damage the cardiovascular system and can potentiate their effects.

4. Some structures of cardiovascular system rather than others are particularly affected by passive smoking because of their functional and anatomical predisposition to be damaged by environmental tobacco smoke components. These sites are those which mainly respond to thrombogenic (hypercoagulability) or atherosclerotic stimuli as well as those intracellular components with elevated metabolism RNA-dependent.
5. Different types of damage are caused by passive smoking exposure on cardiovascular system. One can observe a functional damage that usually follows acute exposure. Endothelial dysfunction, increased catecholamine release, sympathetic system stimulation and impaired cardiac performance tested by exercise stress testing are the functional consequence of acute exposure. A clinical damage characterized mainly by appearance or impairment of clinical signs of ischemic heart and/or cerebrovascular disease occurs usually after chronic exposure or acute exposure of subjects chronically exposed. Anatomical damage, characterized by structural alterations of the heart and blood vessels particularly related to a progression of atherosclerotic lesions with plaque formation especially in coronary and carotid arteries is the final step of passive smoking exposure.
6. Changes in lipid metabolism with increased levels of LDL-cholesterol and decrease in HDL-cholesterol characterize exposure to passive smoking, this pattern has been well-described, particularly in children living with smoker relatives. Also those hemostatic parameters related to coagulation-fibrinolysis cascade activate via thrombi formation together with platelet aggregation and adhesiveness.
7. A large series of epidemiological large-scale studies and metanalyses in humans identify an increased risk of both fatal and nonfatal events following passive smoking exposure due to the presence of coronary heart disease as an underlying disease or stroke. No possibility exists to establish if an intercurrent event will be fatal or nonfatal. Moreover, experimental animal studies demonstrate, with no doubt, that passive smoking causes anatomical and ultrastructural alterations, which are always present although with a different degree, of blood vessels and myocardium.
8. Special categories like women, children and elderly subjects may respond with different characteristics to smoking exposure. That might be due to physiological constellation typical of these people in the different ages of their life.
9. Since exposure to passive smoking leads to cardiovascular alterations constantly, passive smoking must be considered an etiologic with a binding cause-effect more than a risk factor of cardiovascular pathology.
10. Finally, the theorem of Leone, as described in preface, defined carefully the type of alterations caused by both active and passive smoking on cardiovascular system. Theorem has been formulated as follows: "Active smoking injures the cardiovascular system chronically, causing structural lesions, which become, in the long run, irreversible alterations mainly related to coronary atherosclerosis. In contrast, passive smoking causes transiently impaired cardiac performance which may be considerably

more harmful for those people with established ischemic heart disease". This theorem had been formulated on 1995. As one can see by reading this book, in the decade after further studies have demonstrated, undoubtedly, the same final alterations for cardiovascular system as a consequence of either active smoking or chronic exposure to passive smoking possible characteristics of irreversibility, even when passive smoking is the responsible factor.

This decalogue must accompany till today our knowledge on the effects of passive smoking on heart and blood vessels, keeping in mind that more and more studies tend to identify newer cardiovascular alterations due to negative effects of passive smoking, as the studies on endothelial progenitor circulating cells or intracellular enzyme chains of myocardium show susceptible to cause further possible increase in damage.

INDEX

A

B

C

D

E

F

G

H

K

L

M

Q

R

S

T

U

V

W

X

Y